Otolaryngology for the Internist

Guest Editor

MATTHEW W. RYAN, MD

MEDICAL CLINICS
OF NORTH AMERICA

www.medical.theclinics.com

September 2010 • Volume 94 • Number 5

SAUNDERS an imprint of ELSEVIER, Inc.

W.B. SAUNDERS COMPANY
A Division of Elsevier Inc.

1600 John F. Kennedy Boulevard • Suite 1800 • Philadelphia, Pennsylvania 19103-2899

http://www.theclinics.com

MEDICAL CLINICS OF NORTH AMERICA Volume 94, Number 5
September 2010 ISSN 0025-7125, ISBN-13: 978-1-4377-2465-3

Editor: Rachel Glover
Developmental Editor: Jessica Demetriou

Medical Clinics of North America (ISSN 0025-7125) is published bimonthly by Elsevier Inc., 360 Park Avenue South, New York, NY 10010-1710. Months of issue are January, March, May, July, September, and November. Periodicals postage paid at New York, NY, and additional mailing offices. Subscription prices are USD 204 per year for US individuals, USD 361 per year for US institutions, USD 105 per year for US students, USD 259 per year for Canadian individuals, USD 469 per year for Canadian institutions, USD 165 per year for Canadian students, USD 314 per year for international individuals, USD 469 per year for international institutions and USD 165 per year for international students. To receive student/resident rate, orders must be accompanied by name of affiliated institution, date of term, and the *signature* of program/residency coordinator on institution letterhead. Orders will be billed at individual rate until proof of status is received. Foreign air speed delivery is included in all *Clinics* subscription prices. All prices are subject to change without notice. **POSTMASTER:** Send address changes to *Medical Clinics of North America*, Elsevier Health Sciences Division, Subscription Customer Service, 3251 Riverport Lane, Maryland Heights, MO 63043. **Customer Service: Telephone: 1-800-654-2452** (U.S. and Canada); **1-314-447-8871** (outside U.S. and Canada). **Fax: 1-314-447-8029. E-mail: journalscustomerservice-usa@elsevier.com** (for print support); **journalsonlinesupport-usa@ elsevier.com** (for online support).

Reprints. For copies of 100 or more of articles in this publication, please contact the Commercial Reprints Department, Elsevier Inc., 360 Park Avenue South, New York, NY 10010-1710. Tel.: 212-633-3812; Fax: 212-462-1935; E-mail: reprints@elsevier.com.

Medical Clinics of North America is also published in Spanish by McGraw-Hill Interamericana Editores S. A., P.O. Box 5-237, 06500 Mexico, D.F., Mexico.

Medical Clinics of North America is covered in *MEDLINE/PubMed (Index Medicus), Current Contents, ASCA, Excerpta Medica, Science Citation Index,* and *ISI/BIOMED.*

Printed in the United States of America.

GOAL STATEMENT
The goal of *Medical Clinics of North America* is to keep practicing physicians up to date with current clinical practice by providing timely articles reviewing the state of the art in patient care.

ACCREDITATION
The *Medical Clinics of North America* is planned and implemented in accordance with the Essential Areas and Policies of the Accreditation Council for Continuing Medical Education (ACCME) through the joint sponsorship of the University of Virginia School of Medicine and Elsevier. The University of Virginia School of Medicine is accredited by the ACCME to provide continuing medical education for physicians.

The University of Virginia School of Medicine designates this educational activity for a maximum of 15 *AMA PRA Category 1 Credits*™ for each issue, 90 credits per year. Physicians should only claim credit commensurate with the extent of their participation in the activity.

The American Medical Association has determined that physicians not licensed in the US who participate in this CME activity are eligible for a maximum of 15 *AMA PRA Category 1 Credits*™ for each issue, 90 credits per year.

Credit can be earned by reading the text material, taking the CME examination online at http://www.theclinics.com/home/cme, and completing the evaluation. After taking the test, you will be required to review any and all incorrect answers. Following completion of the test and evaluation, your credit will be awarded and you may print your certificate.

FACULTY DISCLOSURE/CONFLICT OF INTEREST
The University of Virginia School of Medicine, as an ACCME accredited provider, endorses and strives to comply with the Accreditation Council for Continuing Medical Education (ACCME) Standards of Commercial Support, Commonwealth of Virginia statutes, University of Virginia policies and procedures, and associated federal and private regulations and guidelines on the need for disclosure and monitoring of proprietary and financial interests that may affect the scientific integrity and balance of content delivered in continuing medical education activities under our auspices.

The University of Virginia School of Medicine requires that all CME activities accredited through this institution be developed independently and be scientifically rigorous, balanced and objective in the presentation/discussion of its content, theories and practices.

All authors/editors participating in an accredited CME activity are expected to disclose to the readers relevant financial relationships with commercial entities occurring within the past 12 months (such as grants or research support, employee, consultant, stock holder, member of speakers bureau, etc.). The University of Virginia School of Medicine will employ appropriate mechanisms to resolve potential conflicts of interest to maintain the standards of fair and balanced education to the reader. Questions about specific strategies can be directed to the Office of Continuing Medical Education, University of Virginia School of Medicine, Charlottesville, Virginia.

The faculty and staff of the University of Virginia Office of Continuing Medical Education have no financial affiliations to disclose.

The authors/editors listed below have identified no professional or financial affiliations for themselves or their spouse/partner:
Jimmy J. Brown, MD, DDS; Neal W. Burkhalter, MD; Teresa V. Chan, MD; Emily Crozier, MD; Christine B. Franzese, MD; Rachel Glover (Acquisitions Editor); Gina D. Jefferson, MD; Ted Mau, MD, PhD; Matthew O. Miller, MD; Ryan E. Neilan, MD; Tara L. Rosenberg, MD; Baran D. Sumer, MD; Seckin O. Ulualp, MD; and Andrew Wolf, MD (Test Author).

The authors/editors listed below identified the following professional or financial affiliations for themselves or their spouse/partner:
Brandon Isaacson, MD is on the Speakers' Bureau for Medtronic Midas Rex Institute.
Joe Walter Kutz Jr, MD is an industry funded research/investigator for Otonomy.
R. Peter Manes, MD is an industry funded research/investigator for MedInvent.
Peter S. Roland, MD is employed by Alcon, and is on the Advisory Committee/Board for Alcon, Med El, and Cochlear.
Matthew W. Ryan, MD (Guest Editor) is on the Speakers' Bureau for Merck.

Disclosure of Discussion of Non-FDA Approved Uses for Pharmaceutical Products and/or Medical Devices.
The University of Virginia School of Medicine, as an ACCME provider, requires that all faculty presenters identify and disclose any off-label uses for pharmaceutical and medical device products. The University of Virginia School of Medicine recommends that each physician fully review all the available data on new products or procedures prior to clinical use.

TO ENROLL
To enroll in the Medical Clinics of North America Continuing Medical Education program, call customer service at 1-800-654-2452 or visit us online at http://www.theclinics.com/home/cme. The CME program is available to subscribers for an additional fee of USD 228.

THE CLINICS ARE NOW AVAILABLE ONLINE!

Access your subscription at:
www.theclinics.com

Contributors

GUEST EDITOR

MATTHEW W. RYAN, MD
Assistant Professor, Department of Otolaryngology–Head and Neck Surgery, University
of Texas Southwestern Medical Center, Dallas, Texas

AUTHORS

JIMMY J. BROWN, MD, DDS, FACS
Professor, Department of Otolaryngology–Head and Neck Surgery, Medical College
of Georgia, Augusta, Georgia

NEAL W. BURKHALTER, MD
Department of Otolaryngology and Communicative Sciences, University of Mississlppi
Medical Center, Jackson, Mississippi

TERESA V. CHAN, MD
Assistant Professor, Department of Otolaryngology–Head and Neck Surgery, University
of Texas Southwestern Medical Center, Dallas, Texas

EMILY CROZIER, MD
Department of Otolaryngology–Head and Neck Surgery, University of Texas
Southwestern Medical Center, Dallas, Texas

CHRISTINE B. FRANZESE, MD
Associate Professor; Residency Program Director, Department of Otolaryngology and
Communicative Sciences, University of Mississippi Medical Center, Jackson, Mississippi

BRANDON ISAACSON, MD, FACS
Assistant Professor, Department of Otolaryngology–Head and Neck Surgery, University
of Texas Southwestern Medical Center, Dallas, Texas

GINA D. JEFFERSON, MD
Assistant Professor, Department of Otolaryngology and Communicative Sciences,
University of Mississippi Medical Center, Jackson, Mississippi

JOE WALTER KUTZ Jr, MD
Assistant Professor, Department of Otolaryngology–Head and Neck Surgery, University
of Texas Southwestern Medical Center, Dallas, Texas

R. PETER MANES, MD
Clinical Instructor, Department of Otolaryngology–Head and Neck Surgery, University
of Texas Southwestern Medical Center, Dallas, Texas

TED MAU, MD, PhD
Assistant Professor, Clinical Center for Voice Care, Department of Otolaryngology–Head
and Neck Surgery, University of Texas Southwestern Medical Center, Dallas, Texas

MATTHEW C. MILLER, MD
Assistant Professor of Head and Neck Oncologic and Microvascular Reconstructive Surgery, Department of Otolaryngology–Head and Neck Surgery, University of Rochester Medical Center, Rochester, New York

RYAN E. NEILAN, MD
Department of Otolaryngology–Head and Neck Surgery, University of Texas Southwestern Medical Center, Dallas, Texas

PETER S. ROLAND, MD
Professor and Chairman, Department of Otolaryngology–Head and Neck Surgery, Southwestern Medical Center, Dallas, Texas

TARA L. ROSENBERG, MD
Post-Graduate Resident Physician, Department of Otolaryngology and Communicative Sciences, University of Mississippi Medical Center, Jackson, Mississippi

MATTHEW W. RYAN, MD
Assistant Professor, Department of Otolaryngology–Head and Neck Surgery, University of Texas Southwestern Medical Center, Dallas, Texas

BARAN D. SUMER, MD
Assistant Professor, Department of Otolaryngology–Head and Neck Surgery, University of Texas Southwestern Medical Center, Dallas, Texas

SECKIN O. ULUALP, MD
Assistant Professor, Department of Otolaryngology–Head and Neck Surgery, University of Texas Southwestern Medical Center, Dallas, Texas

Contents

The patient with "sinus" is common. However, an accurate diagnosis for a patient's sinus complaints may be elusive. The diagnostic uncertainty with these patients is a result of nonspecific symptoms, subtle or absent physical examination findings, and limited diagnostic testing options. Rhinitis should be distinguished from sinusitis. In acute illness, viral upper respiratory tract infection should be distinguished from acute bacterial sinusitis. For patients with chronic sinus symptoms, objective evidence of paranasal sinus inflammation should be confirmed before labeling the patient with chronic sinusitis.

Allergic disease affects a sizeable percentage of the general population, has a significant impact on patient quality of life, and exerts a significant financial burden on society. Atopic symptoms from inhalant allergens are among the most frequent complaints in outpatient medical visits. Key history and physical examination findings help to distinguish allergic rhinitis from other forms of chronic rhinosinusitis. Diagnostic testing may not be necessary unless immunotherapy is contemplated.

Epistaxis is a common clinical problem often seen by primary care physicians. This can be caused by multiple factors, each of which should be explored to treat the epistaxis and prevent recurrences. In this article, etiologies and methods of evaluation for the patient with epistaxis are discussed. Treatment strategies are outlined in a stepwise fashion, as are recommendations for situations requiring referral to an otolaryngologist.

Postnasal drip (PND) is a common clinical complaint, yet its physiologic basis and appropriate treatment have been inadequately addressed in the medical literature. PND may be caused by a variety of conditions involving the nose and throat. Often, the symptom is not caused by actual secretions draining from the nose into the pharynx. In many instances, no definitive cause can be identified. Empiric treatment for PND symptoms should be guided by associated symptoms that suggest either a sinonasal cause or gastroesophageal reflux. Rarely, PND may be a symptom of a serious process such as a mass lesion in the pharynx or a malignancy and thus referral to an otolaryngologist is appropriate if symptoms are persistent, unexplainable, or associated with warning signs of malignancy.

loss markedly increases with advancing age. The differential diagnosis for patients presenting with hearing loss is extensive, but can often be narrowed with a directed hearing history and physical examination. The severity of the hearing loss may warrant additional diagnostic studies, including audiometry, and possible imaging in selected cases. Hearing aids, assistive listening devices, middle ear surgery, and cochlear implantation are potential therapeutic options available to patients depending on the type and severity of the hearing loss.

Joe Walter Kutz Jr

The dizzy patient often presents a challenge to the physician. The history is the most important component of the evaluation of the dizzy patient and often allows the cause of the dizziness to be categorized as peripheral or central. Peripheral causes include benign paroxysmal positional vertigo, Meniere's disease, and vestibular neuritis. Central causes include migraine-associated dizziness, postconcussion syndromes, cerebrovascular disease, and multiple sclerosis. Treatment depends on the cause of the dizziness and may include dietary modifications, diuretics, vestibular suppressants, vestibular rehabilitation, or surgical intervention.

Matthew C. Miller

Nodular thyroid disease is common in the United States and throughout the world. Although most thyroid nodules are benign in nature, certain clinical, radiographic, and cytologic features are associated with an increased risk of malignancy. A clear understanding of these risk factors assists in the decision-making process when evaluating a patient with a thyroid nodule. It is this process that ultimately determines whether or not a patient is referred for surgery. This article provides a framework for clinicians to risk-stratify and appropriately manage patients with thyroid nodules.

Tara L. Rosenberg, Jimmy J. Brown, and Gina D. Jefferson

The objective of this article is to provide the internist with general considerations when confronted with an adult patient presenting with a neck mass. A thorough gathering of historical information and a complete physical examination are crucial in developing a differential diagnosis for these patients. Specifically, the location of the mass, its time of onset, and duration are important because of the high likelihood of neoplastic processes in patients older than 40 years. The young adult patient has an increased incidence of inflammatory, congenital, and traumatic processes as causes of their neck mass, but again, neoplasms are not out of the realm of possibility. Judicious use of imaging studies, namely computed tomography scanning with contrast, is a valuable adjunct to the physical examination. Other than infectious etiology, referral to an otolaryngologist is frequently warranted to obtain a definitive diagnosis for the development of an appropriate treatment plan, which is predominantly surgical.

> Early detection of upper aerodigestive tract cancer improves prognosis. The primary care physician plays an important role in early detection of these cancers. Most upper aerodigestive tract cancers are squamous cell carcinomas that are linked to tobacco, alcohol, or human papillomavirus exposure. These cancers produce nonspecific symptoms; thus, any persistent oral cavity lesion or neck mass or other unexplainable ear, nose, and throat symptoms should prompt an evaluation for malignancy. Although overall survival has not improved, nonsurgical treatment approaches have led to higher rates of organ preservation and rehabilitation after treatment has improved the quality of life of survivors.

> Obstructive sleep apnea (OSA) may be associated with myriad clinical consequences such as increased risk of systemic hypertension, coronary vascular disease, congestive heart failure, cerebrovascular disease, glucose intolerance, impotence, obesity, pulmonary hypertension, gastroesophageal reflux, and impaired concentration. Nonetheless, OSA remains undiagnosed in 82% of men and 93% of women with the condition. Early identification and treatment of OSA provides significant relief for individuals, prevents complications of OSA, and reduces overall health care costs. Better understanding of the pathogenesis, risk factors, diagnosis, and treatment of OSA has the potential to improve early recognition of OSA and prevention of adverse effects on the individual and society.

Preface

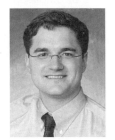

Matthew W. Ryan, MD
Guest Editor

Acute and chronic conditions of the ear, nose, throat, and related head and neck structures are common reasons for outpatient medical visits. These conditions, and the symptoms they cause, can be trivial and mundane or may be debilitating with profound impacts on quality of life. They may be self-limiting and only require supportive care. On the other hand, as pointed out in the articles in this issue of the *Medical Clinics of North America*, seemingly benign symptoms may be the first clues to a serious and life-threatening condition. General internists stand at the frontline of the effort to make an early diagnosis that has an impact on treatment outcome. The diagnosis and management of these head and neck conditions can be a challenge for general internists (or otolaryngology specialists for that matter), and significant judgment is required to discern the significance of a patient's complaints, begin treatment despite diagnostic uncertainty, and use diagnostic testing in a cost-effective manner.

For ambulatory otolaryngology problems, the history and physical examination are often all that is required to render an accurate diagnosis and begin treatment. Laboratory tests are not usually necessary. One of my attractions to otolaryngology as a career field derived from the primacy of physical examination as a diagnostic tool. Unfortunately, general internists do not often possess the equipment that enables a detailed physical examination of the head and neck. In the absence of an operating microscope and flexible and rigid endoscopes, generalists must be even more skilled in analyzing a patient's history and in using other diagnostic tools, such as imaging.

Residency training for internists may not significantly address the head and neck problems that are common in ambulatory medical practice. Thus, a goal of this issue is to share the otolaryngologist's perspective on the evaluation and management of patients with common head and neck problems. Each article is oriented toward a specific chief complaint, with diagnostic and treatment strategies that are primarily practical in nature. A variety of texts are available that provide interested readers with a more encyclopedic description of the multiple pathologies that affect the head and neck. Finally, we have endeavored to identify red flags that suggest a referral when specialty care is needed, and we have included an article that provides an

Med Clin N Am 94 (2010) xi–xii
doi:10.1016/j.mcna.2010.05.012
0025-7125/10/$ – see front matter © 2010 Elsevier Inc. All rights reserved.

update on the diagnosis and treatment of upper aerodigestive tract malignancy. It is hoped that the contents of this issue provide practicing general internists with some novel insights and strategies that can be used in the management of outpatients who present with head and neck symptoms.

Matthew W. Ryan, MD
Department of Otolaryngology–Head and Neck Surgery
University of Texas Southwestern Medical Center
5323 Harry Hines Boulevard
Dallas, TX 75390-9035, USA

E-mail address:
Matthew.ryan@utsouthwestern.edu

Evaluation and Management of the Patient with "Sinus"

Matthew W. Ryan, MD

KEYWORDS

• Sinus • Sinusitis • Acute sinusitis • Chronic sinusitis
• Rhinosinusitis

THE TROUBLESOME PATIENT WITH SINUS COMPLAINTS

Sinus complaints are common presenting symptoms in both general and specialty practice. An estimated 20% of outpatient antibiotic prescriptions in the United States can be attributed to acute or chronic sinusitis.[1] Allergic rhinitis is estimated to affect 10% to 30% of the US population,[2] and adults experience approximately 4 acute viral upper respiratory tract infections (URTIs) per year.[3] Conventional wisdom holds that approximately 0.5% to 2% of viral URTIs will evolve into an acute bacterial sinusitis.[3] Some individuals may be prone to develop recurrent upper respiratory infections because of environmental exposures, comorbid conditions such as allergic rhinitis, and rarely, immunodeficiency.[4] The role of sinonasal anatomic deformity, cigarette smoking, and air pollution as causative factors for upper respiratory illness is likely but unproven. In some instances, no predisposing factors can be identified, and some individuals may be prone to seek medical care for simple URTIs that would be tolerated by most of the population.

Unlike many other conditions, patients with sinonasal symptoms often present complaining of a diagnosis. The patients may complain of sinus, by which they mean sinusitis, or allergies by which they mean allergic rhinitis. This self-diagnosis is often incorrect, and it becomes the physician's responsibility to determine the underlying process. This tendency toward self-diagnosis is fostered by a general societal awareness of respiratory conditions, the patient's upbringing, personal experiences, and previous medical encounters. It is also likely that ubiquitous advertisement of a variety of over-the-counter sinus medications contributes to patient perceptions and misinterpretation of symptoms.

The patient with sinus challenges the generalist physician to make accurate diagnoses, provide appropriate medical treatment that is also acceptable to the patient, minimize the unnecessary use of antibiotics, and limit overutilization of health care

Department of Otolaryngology, University of Texas Southwestern Medical Center, 5323 Harry Hines Boulevard, Dallas, TX 75390-9035, USA
E-mail address: matthew.ryan@utsouthwestern.edu

Med Clin N Am 94 (2010) 881–890
doi:10.1016/j.mcna.2010.05.013
0025-7125/10/$ – see front matter © 2010 Elsevier Inc. All rights reserved.

system resources. One aim of this article is to confront the lay wisdom of patients about sinus disease and help the clinician develop an effective cost-conscious approach to manage these patients. A more encyclopedic synthesis of available information on rhinitis and sinusitis can be accessed via several well-written guidelines.[2,5]

SYMPTOMS OF SINUS DISEASE ARE OFTEN NONSPECIFIC

Among the frustrations and difficulties that go along with the assessment and treatment of patients with sinonasal complaints, perhaps the most difficult is the process of gathering information that can yield a reliable diagnosis. As discussed later, there are some diagnostic tools to determine the presence of sinus inflammation, but in a primary care setting, the patient's history provides the most useful information.

However, the symptoms of rhinitis and sinusitis can be subtle, absent, or misleading. Symptoms that may be reasonably attributed to sinonasal inflammation include nasal congestion, nasal stuffiness, nasal airway obstruction, a decreased sense of smell and taste, anterior rhinorrhea, postnasal drainage, facial pressure or outright facial pain, cough, fatigue, malaise, ear pressure or fullness, maxillary dental pain, and headache. Detailed questioning of the patient may be required to further elucidate what the patient means when they use these terms. For example, nasal congestion could denote nasal airway obstruction, that is, a perceived increased resistance to nasal airflow. But another patient may use the same term to describe a fullness or pressure sensation within the nasal cavity. So, in addition to acquiring the full list of symptoms that the patient describes, it may also be necessary to clarify the meaning behind commonly used terms.

The symptoms of rhinitis and sinusitis often overlap, and it is increasingly recognized that patients with sinusitis also frequently have inflammation in the nasal cavity, and vice versa. For this reason, the term rhinosinusitis is increasingly used in the literature. Among the symptoms of rhinosinusitis, no single symptom or set of symptoms has been found to be especially sensitive or specific to distinguish acute bacterial sinusitis from other causes of the same symptoms, such as a viral URTI or an exacerbation of allergic or nonallergic rhinitis. In addition, some symptoms such as headache or facial pain, which are commonly attributed to sinus disease by the lay public, may have no relationship to rhinosinusitis. This misperception is reinforced by advertisements for sinus pain remedies. Although midfacial pain may be a prominent symptom of acute maxillary sinusitis, facial pain and headache are not cardinal symptoms of chronic sinonasal inflammatory diseases. Chronic, longstanding, or recurrent headache and facial pain are uncommon symptoms of sinusitis.

PHYSICAL EXAMINATION FINDINGS ARE OFTEN NEITHER SENSITIVE NOR SPECIFIC

Routine physical examination provides little information that is helpful to define the sinonasal inflammatory process that may be causing a patient's symptoms. Nevertheless, a thorough head and neck examination that focuses on the nasal cavity may provide contributory evidence of the underlying disease process. Textbooks on physical diagnosis often describe sinus tenderness, lack of sinus transillumination, or maxillary dental sensitivity as physical findings that support the diagnosis of acute sinusitis. However, these findings are neither sensitive nor specific.

Intranasal examination can determine the presence of inflammatory changes such as mucosal edema or erythema, and abnormal secretions. The classic findings for allergic rhinitis include pale or bluish nasal mucosa with clear secretions. The infected nose is supposedly erythematous with purulent secretions. Although the appearance of the nose is not specific for a particular diagnosis, it does reveal if significant inflammation is present. The visualization of purulent secretions draining from the middle meatus may confirm a clinical diagnosis of acute sinusitis, but such visualization is often impossible with the instrumentation available in most primary care offices. If purulent secretions cannot be visualized with anterior rhinoscopy, a surrogate evaluation is examination of the oropharynx to determine if purulent secretions are draining posteriorly.

Anterior rhinoscopy can be performed with a simple otoscope and is a crucial diagnostic maneuver for the sinus patient. If the nose is significantly congested, 0.5 mL of oxymetazoline nasal spray, loaded into a tuberculin syringe may be sprayed into the nose, and the examination can be repeated in 10 minutes. The goal of this thorough nasal examination is to identify purulent secretions draining from the sinuses, not just secretions stagnating in the nose. A simple viral URTI causes damage to the delicate ciliated respiratory epithelium in the nose. At the same time, inflammation induced by the viral infection will stimulate mucus secretion from goblet cells. This mucus may stagnate in the nose, along with neutrophils. Thus, thick, colored, nasal secretions often develop in the setting of an acute viral URTI, and colored secretions in the nasal cavity are not a specific finding for acute bacterial sinusitis. Also, the apparent absence of purulent secretions in the nose or draining in the oropharynx cannot rule out sinusitis. Therefore, physical examination may not be particularly helpful in many circumstances.

DIAGNOSTIC UNCERTAINTY IS COMMON, AND COMPLICATIONS ARE RARE

Although diagnostic uncertainty is a common problem when patients present to a primary care office with sinonasal complaints, the risk associated with an incorrect diagnosis is low. Rhinosinusitis is mostly a nuisance, and serious complications are rare. Neoplasms and serious disease processes usually cause benign symptoms, but these too are rare. The primary therapeutic goals for sinus patients are symptomatic relief and improvement in quality of life. There are no data to suggest that early antibiotic treatment reduces the occurrence of serious infectious complications (eg, orbital abscess, brain abscess, meningitis) or clinical evolution of an acute process into a chronic process (eg, acute sinusitis evolving to chronic sinusitis). An analysis of placebo-controlled studies of antibiotic treatment for acute bacterial sinusitis failed to find any increased risk for complications from nontreatment with antibiotics.[6] Perhaps the greatest risk of misdiagnosis is the effect that an incorrect diagnosis of a sinus infection has on a patient's future interpretation of upper respiratory symptoms.

There is significant symptomatic overlap between rhinitis and sinusitis. The diagnostic distinction between rhinitis and sinusitis is often challenging, and the differential diagnosis of sinonasal symptoms is quite broad. A distinction between sinusitis and rhinitis is important primarily because sinusitis is treated with antibiotics. Because many medications are useful for both rhinitis and sinusitis (eg, pseudoephedrine, nasal steroid sprays, nasal saline), the clinical distinction of viral versus bacterial disease, and rhinitis versus sinusitis is less important if antibiotic treatment is not being contemplated.

DIAGNOSTIC CATEGORIES FOR SINUSITIS

There are multiple overlapping classification systems for sinusitis. These classification systems do not necessarily correspond with the International Classification of Diseases diagnostic codes. Sinusitis can be classified according to the sinuses involved (maxillary, sphenoid, and so forth), presumed pathogen (viral, bacterial, fungal), or time course of the disease process (acute, subacute, recurrent acute, chronic). Although diagnostic specificity is useful, in practice the most important distinctions are the underlying pathogen and the time course of the disease, because these have treatment implications.

A viral URTI (common cold) is a viral rhinosinusitis, although patients may also have symptoms of conjunctivitis, pharyngitis, laryngitis, or bronchitis. The common cold is most frequently caused by rhinovirus, but also by coronaviruses, parainfluenza virus, respiratory syncytial virus, enteroviruses, and adenoviruses. Although clinical presentation can vary, probably as a result of host and viral factors, typical symptoms include rhinorrhea, nasal congestion and obstruction, facial pain and pressure, headache, sneezing, hoarseness, sore throat, malaise, chills, and cough. Rhinorrhea and sneezing are the most common symptomatic complaints, and headache occurs in 30% of cases.[7] These symptoms overlap significantly with acute bacterial sinusitis and acute exacerbations of allergic or nonallergic rhinitis. That the common cold is really a form of acute viral rhinosinusitis was demonstrated by Gwaltney and colleagues[8] who performed sinus computer tomography (CT) scans on a sample of subjects with the common cold. Most subjects (87%) had findings of sinus inflammation in the maxillary or ethmoid sinuses. So it is now clear that a viral URTI is not just a viral acute rhinitis but actually a form of rhinosinusitis. The common cold is generally self-limited, but antibiotics are prescribed in 30% to 78% of cases that present to a health care provider.[9] In a landmark study by Gwaltney and colleagues[7] the duration of symptoms associated with acute viral URTI, mostly due to rhinovirus, was carefully detailed. The median duration of illness was 7 days, but 25% of subjects had illness for 2 weeks. A small percentage of viral URTIs leads to bacterial sinusitis, otitis media, or exacerbations of asthma and chronic obstructive pulmonary disease. Thus a simple viral URTI can cause significant morbidity.

ACUTE BACTERIAL SINUSITIS

Acute bacterial sinusitis typically develops as a secondary bacterial infection after an acute viral URTI. The pathogens responsible for acute bacterial sinusitis have been well characterized and include *Streptococcus pneumoniae*, *Haemophilus influenzae*, *Moraxella catarrhalis*, and *Staphylococcus aureus*.[10] Rarely, acute maxillary sinusitis can develop from an odontogenic source. A diagnosis of acute bacterial sinusitis may be made in individuals with the symptoms of a viral URTI that have not improved after 10 days or have worsened after 5 to 7 days. In some cases, a clinical diagnosis of acute bacterial sinusitis is appropriate if symptoms are out of proportion to a typical URTI.[6] The gold standard for diagnosing acute bacterial sinusitis is a maxillary sinus puncture with culture of sinus contents. However, because of the discomfort and potential complications of this procedure, antral puncture is rarely performed for clinical purposes. As has been noted, the signs and symptoms of acute bacterial sinusitis do not vary significantly from a viral URTI. Physical examination findings are unreliable, and because a viral URTI will produce inflammatory changes, radiologic studies are not helpful in differentiating viral from bacterial disease.[1] Williams and colleagues[11] performed a prospective study among 247 patients referred for acute sinusitis. Of the 16 symptoms examined, no one symptom was both sensitive and specific. However, regression analysis identified 5 symptoms and signs (maxillary toothache, abnormal transillumination, poor response to decongestants, purulent secretions, and colored nasal discharge by history) that if combined in the same patient, yielded a 92% probability of sinusitis. The findings from this study are often repeated in clinical texts. However, this study did not use correlation with sinus aspirate culture results, nor have other studies that examined signs and symptoms of acute bacterial sinusitis. Thus, consideration of the time course and severity of a patient's symptoms are considered to be the best methods to distinguish viral from bacterial acute rhinosinusitis. Such an approach errs on the side of overtreatment with antibiotics, but a more specific approach entails inordinate cost and potential patient harm.

Acute bacterial sinusitis can cause severe and potentially life-threatening complications including meningitis, orbital cellulitis, orbital abscess or intracranial abscesses. These complications are rare, especially in adult populations. The natural history of untreated cases of acute bacterial sinusitis has not been thoroughly studied. However, in placebo-controlled studies of acute bacterial sinusitis, approximately two-thirds of patients experienced spontaneous symptom resolution.[12] Although theoretically an untreated acute bacterial sinusitis can evolve into chronic sinusitis, the role of acute sinusitis in the pathogenesis of chronic sinus disease is unclear, and antibiotic trials for acute sinusitis have not examined this question.

Chronic sinusitis is a condition that continues to be a source of confusion and controversy. The terms chronic sinusitis and chronic rhinosinusitis (CRS) are now used interchangeably to refer to a group of disorders that are characterized by inflammation of the nasal and paranasal sinus mucosa over a prolonged period of time (>12 weeks), with accompanying clinical signs and symptoms.[13] This definition allows for a variety of underlying pathophysiologic processes, extrinsic triggers, and clinical phenotypes. Chronic sinusitis can be categorized according to the presence or absence of nasal polyps,[5] but a widely accepted and useful classification system for the various subtypes of chronic sinusitis remains elusive.

The diagnosis of chronic sinusitis is as problematic as the accurate diagnosis of acute bacterial sinusitis. The symptoms of chronic sinusitis are similar to acute sinusitis (in some ways, chronic sinusitis is clinically a cold that will not go away). However, there is significant symptomatic overlap between chronic rhinitis and chronic sinusitis. Physical examination abnormalities that are detectable on a routine head and neck examination may be absent in chronic sinusitis. Widespread use of sinus imaging is costly, and most generalists who treat chronic sinusitis do not use nasal endoscopy. For these reasons, a consensus statement published in 1997 recommended that the clinical diagnosis of chronic sinusitis rely primarily on the patient's history, using a set of major and minor clinical factors to make the diagnosis.[13] However, when this approach was evaluated in clinical studies that combined symptomatic history with objective evaluation for sinus inflammation (nasal endoscopy, sinus CT), it was revealed that this approach overdiagnosed chronic sinusitis in about 50% of cases.[14] A recent clinical practice guideline recommends that the diagnosis of chronic sinusitis should be accompanied by objective evidence of paranasal sinus inflammation. This objective evidence can be obtained via radiologic studies or by rhinoscopy that shows purulent mucus, edema, or polyps in the middle meatus.[4] The added costs of radiography or nasal endoscopy are offset by the savings from a reduction in unnecessary treatment. Thus, a clinical diagnosis of chronic sinusitis should no longer rely on symptoms alone.

A variety of microorganisms can be cultured from the nose and paranasal sinuses of patients with chronic sinusitis. However, there is significant room for debate regarding whether the presence of these microorganisms indicates a causative role in the patient's inflammatory disease. Traditionally, bacteria have been assumed to be the causative organisms in chronic sinusitis, and antibiotic therapy is commonly used to treat the disease. Microbiologic studies have demonstrated that the bacteriology of chronic sinusitis is different from acute bacterial sinusitis; in chronic sinusitis, anerobes and gram-negative organisms are frequently present. Polymicrobial involvement is common in chronic sinusitis, and the bacteriology changes in patients who have previously undergone sinus surgery.[10] Some bacteria in the paranasal sinuses may form biofilms that are refractory to eradication with standard antimicrobial therapy. However, chronic sinusitis is not necessarily an infectious disease, and microorganisms that colonize the nose and paranasal sinuses may stimulate inflammation without tissue invasion.[5] Recent attention has focused on the possible role that fungi or enterotoxin-producing staphylococci may play as extrinsic factors that trigger the inflammation observed in chronic sinusitis. These theories have treatment implications that remain to be resolved.

DIAGNOSTIC TOOLS FOR SINUSITIS

Besides the history and physical examination, the primary diagnostic aids for sinusitis are radiologic imaging and nasal endoscopy. Because viral URTIs cause inflammatory changes within the paranasal sinuses, radiographic imaging for the diagnosis of acute bacterial sinusitis is not appropriate unless a complication or alternative diagnosis is suspected (such as a malignancy, or facial pain not caused by sinusitis).[4] Examples of complications that warrant imaging include orbital, intracranial, or facial soft tissue spread of infection. If imaging is considered, CT is preferred over plain films or magnetic resonance imaging (MRI) because of improved visualization of the paranasal sinus anatomy. Evaluation of abscess formation requires intravenous contrast, and if intracranial involvement is suspected, MRI is appropriate.[4] In general, adjunctive testing is neither necessary nor appropriate in most cases of acute rhinosinusitis.

The diagnosis of chronic sinusitis requires confirmation of paranasal sinus inflammation by examination or radiography. The differential diagnoses for CRS symptoms include allergic and nonallergic rhinitis, nasal septal deviation, and various other causes of headache and facial pain. Reliance on history alone has been shown to be an unreliable means to distinguish chronic sinusitis from these other possibilities. Routine anterior rhinoscopy is often insufficient because of poor visualization. Nasal endoscopy that demonstrates purulent drainage, polyps, or edema in the middle meatus or sphenoethmoidal recess is sufficient to make the diagnosis. In addition, endoscopy facilitates culture-directed antibiotic treatment because purulent exudates draining from the sinuses can be sampled with minimal morbidity. However, because endoscopic tools and training are not widely available in primary care settings, radiologic imaging is a primary diagnostic modality for chronic sinusitis.

A noncontrasted CT of the sinuses is considered the gold standard imaging test for the diagnosis of chronic sinusitis.[4] CT can assess the patency of sinus outflow tracts, identify fluid collections and mucosal thickening within the paranasal sinuses, and occasionally reveal tumors, masses, or mucoceles that are not suspected from the clinical history. In addition, CT may identify anatomic abnormalities that are predisposing to sinus outflow tract obstruction. As a diagnostic modality, CT is not foolproof. Imaging may fail to detect small polyps and mucus recirculation phenomena. In addition, sinus abnormalities are frequently present despite a lack of chronic sinusitis symptoms.[15] Multiple studies have shown that the extent of CT abnormalities does not correlate with symptom burden.[16] CT is the best diagnostic tool for chronic sinusitis, but as with any diagnostic test the imaging findings must be correlated with the patient's history. A variety of other diagnostic tests may be used in select circumstances for patients with acute or chronic sinusitis including cystic fibrosis testing, allergy tests, and immunologic evaluation. However, a discussion of these testing modalities is outside of the scope of this article.

MEDICAL TREATMENT

Medical treatment for the patient with sinus should be directed toward the underlying diagnosis and pathophysiologic process. A variety of comprehensive clinical practice guidelines and practice parameters for the treatment of rhinitis and acute sinusitis have been developed from exhaustive reviews of the literature, and these provide useful guidance for appropriate medical treatment.[2,4,12] However, many patients with sinus do not have a history and examination that fits into a neat diagnostic category. For these individuals a symptom-based treatment approach is appropriate, and the history should be revisited in an attempt to identify the primary symptoms as well as aggravating and relieving factors for these symptoms. These patients can be difficult to treat, but positive treatment outcomes can result from an approach that educates patients about the physiologic basis for their symptoms and establishes a commitment to a patient search for beneficial measures. It is surprising how frequently patients will self-treat in an incorrect fashion (eg, taking antihistamines for facial pain.) The physician is well positioned to recommend more appropriate medical intervention and monitor symptomatic improvement.

Medical treatment of acute bacterial sinusitis has been thoroughly studied. The best established treatment for acute bacterial sinusitis is a 7 to 10 days course of oral antibiotics, although some antibiotics have demonstrated benefit with shorter courses of therapy. Despite the increase in antibiotic resistance and the known prevalence of β-lactamase–producing organisms, amoxicillin and trimethoprim/sulfamethoxazole are still often recommended as first-line therapy for acute sinusitis.[10,12] Early treatment failure, severity of symptoms, and likelihood of resistant organisms are cited as reasons to consider β-lactamase–resistant or broader spectrum antibiotics. A recent body of randomized trials has also demonstrated that nasal steroid sprays reduce symptom severity and hasten symptom resolution in the setting of acute sinusitis.[17] Therefore, consideration should be given to the use of a nasal steroid spray in addition to an antibiotic. Other symptomatic measures such as oral and topical nasal decongestants, analgesics, and nasal saline are believed to be helpful in acute sinusitis despite a lack of clinical trials.

The appropriate medical management of chronic sinusitis has not been thoroughly studied. The medical management of chronic sinusitis typically includes antibiotics, antiinflammatory agents, and saline lavage. Usually, broad-spectrum antibiotic therapy is recommended that covers aerobic and anerobic organisms, and β-lactamase producers.[10] An antibiotic course of 4 to 8 weeks is recommended. Antiinflammatory medication consists of a brief course of systemic corticosteroid along with prolonged use of a topical nasal steroid spray. Uncontrolled cohort studies have shown that this approach results in significant symptomatic improvement in most patients.[18]

There is a paucity of randomized trials for the treatment of chronic sinusitis, and there are no accepted clinical practice guidelines for the medical management of chronic sinusitis. The lack of clinical trial data and treatment guidance is a direct result of difficulty in defining the disease process and categorizing its subtypes. As mentioned previously, chronic sinusitis is a broad term that includes multiple pathophysiologic processes that result in chronic sinus inflammation. Traditional treatment approaches have tended to lump all chronic sinusitis together.

One dominant working model has assumed that chronic sinusitis is an intense bacterial sinusitis that evolves from an initial acute bacterial sinusitis. Explanations for the persistence of this bacterial infection have included sinus outflow tract obstruction, bacterial osteitis, and biofilm formation. In many cases of chronic sinusitis these factors may be important. However, appropriately powered placebo-controlled trials of oral antibiotic treatment for chronic sinusitis have not been performed. A single randomized placebo-controlled study of low-dose roxithromycin for nonpolypoid CRS showed equivocal results.[19] A few topical antibiotic trials have been performed, but the results were essentially negative.[20,21] Other approaches, such as the use of intravenous antibiotics have not been studied in any sort of controlled trial. Thus, the antibiotic treatment of chronic sinusitis is still poorly substantiated and more placebo-controlled trials are needed.

There is a much stronger body of clinical evidence for the treatment of CRS with nasal polyps. Topical nasal steroid sprays as well as oral steroids have been shown via randomized placebo-controlled trials to reduce nasal polyp size and reduce symptoms.[22,23] Antibiotics have not been appropriately studied in polypoid CRS, but multiple trials have examined the efficacy of topical amphotericin B, in a test of the fungal hypothesis. These studies have not shown any significant clinical benefit, and topical amphotericin B is not recommended for the treatment of chronic sinusitis with nasal polyps.[24–26] Although antiinflammatory agents like corticosteroids seem to be beneficial for chronic sinusitis with nasal polyps, there is no standard dosing regimen. Brief courses of systemic steroids are recommended because of their long-term toxicities. Topical nasal steroids do seem to have a dose-response effect, and given their low bioavailability, increasing doses of topical steroids are preferred over systemic administration.

INDICATIONS FOR REFERRAL

The patient with sinus will frequently benefit from consultation with an otolaryngologist. Absolute indications for referral include complications from sinusitis, suspected neoplasm, mucocele, or fungal sinusitis. However, the most common indications for referral include persistent symptoms despite apparently appropriate medical treatment, atypical symptoms, anatomic abnormalities, recurrent sinusitis, and massive nasal polyposis. Surgery is frequently used for patients with anatomic deformity, inadequate improvement with medical therapy, or conditions that are not amenable to medical therapy (eg, deviated septum, mucocele) Although most rhinosinusitis is a medical disease, some patients will only benefit from a combination of medical and surgical approaches. Consultation with an otolaryngologist may permit a more precise diagnosis and treatment of the underlying cause of the sinus complaints.

SUMMARY

The patient with sinus can be difficult to treat for a variety of reasons. Although the patient's history is the most important aspect of diagnosis, this history also provides nonspecific information. There is considerable overlap between rhinitis and sinusitis symptoms, and patients may inappropriately ascribe their symptoms to sinus disease. Precise diagnostic tools are lacking for acute illness, and the best medical management approach for patients with chronic sinusitis is poorly defined. In cases of diagnostic uncertainty or poor treatment response, consultation with an otolaryngologist is appropriate.

REFERENCES

1. Marple BF, Brunton S, Ferguson BJ. Acute bacterial rhinosinusitis: a review of US treatment guidelines. Otolaryngol Head Neck Surg 2006;135:341–8.

2. Wallace DV, Dykewicz MS, Bernstein DI, et al. The diagnosis and management of rhinitis: an updated practice parameter. J Allergy Clin Immunol 2008;122:S1–84.
3. Gwaltney JM, Wiesinger BA, Patrie JT. Acute community-acquired bacterial sinusitis: the value of antimicrobial treatment and the natural history. Clin Infect Dis 2004;38:227–33.
4. Rosenfeld RM, Andes D, Bhattacharyya N, et al. Clinical practice guideline: adult sinusitis. Otolaryngol Head Neck Surg 2007;137:S1–31.
5. Meltzer EO, Hamilos DL, Hadley JA, et al. Rhinosinusitis: establishing definitions for clinical research and patient care. Otolaryngol Head Neck Surg 2004;131:S1–62.
6. Lau J, Zucker D, Engels EA, et al. Diagnosis and treatment of acute bacterial rhinosinusitis. Evidence report/technology assessment no. 9 (contract 290-97-0019 to the New England Medical Center). Rockville (MD): Agency for Health Care Policy and Research; 1999.
7. Gwaltney JM, Hendley JO, Simon G, et al. Rhinovirus infections in an industrial population. JAMA 1967;202(6):158–64.
8. Gwaltney JM, Phillips CD, Miller RD, et al. Computed tomography study of the common cold. N Engl J Med 1994;330:25–30.
9. Larson EL. Warned, but not well armed: preventing viral upper respiratory infections in households. Public Health Nurs 2007;24(1):48–59.
10. Brook I. Microbiology and antimicrobial management of sinusitis. J Laryngol Otol 2005;119:251–8.
11. Williams JW, Simel DL, Roberts L, et al. Clinical evaluation for sinusitis: making the diagnosis by history and physical examination. Ann Intern Med 1992;117:705–10.
12. Ip S, Fu L, Balk E, et al. Update on acute bacterial rhinosinusitis. Evidence report/technology assessment no. 124 (prepared by Tufts-New England Medical Center Evidence-based Practice Center under contract no. 290-02-0022). AHRQ publication no. 05-E020-2. Rockville (MD): Agency for Healthcare Research and Quality; 2005.
13. Lanza DC, Kennedy DW. Adult rhinosinusitis defined. Otolaryngol Head Neck Surg 1997;117:S1–7.
14. Stankiewicz JA, Chow JM. Nasal endoscopy and the definition and diagnosis of chronic rhinosinusitis. Otolaryngol Head Neck Surg 2002;126:623–7.
15. Ashraf N, Bhattacharyya N. Determination of the "incidental" Lund score for the staging of chronic rhinosinusitis. Otolaryngol Head Neck Surg 2001;125:483–6.
16. Basu S, Georgalas C, Kumar BN, et al. Correlation between symptoms and radiological findings in patients with chronic rhinosinusitis: an evaluation study using the Sinonasal Assessment Questionnaire and Lund-Mackay grading system. Eur Arch Otorhinolaryngol 2005;262:751–4.
17. Zalmanovici A. Yaphe J. Intranasal steroids for acute sinusitis. Cochrane Database Syst 2009;4:CD005149.
18. Subramanian HN, Schechtman KB, Hamilos DL. A retrospective analysis of treatment outcomes and time to relapse after intensive medical treatment for chronic sinusitis. Am J Rhinol 2002;16:303–12.
19. Wallwork B, Coman W, Mackay-Sim A, et al. A double-blind, randomized, placebo-controlled trial of macrolide in the treatment of chronic rhinosinusitis. Laryngoscope 2006;116:189–93.
20. Derosier MY, Salas-Prato M. Treatment of chronic rhinosinusitis refractory to other treatments with topical antibiotic therapy delivered by means of a large-particle

nebulizer: results of a controlled trial. Otolaryngol Head Neck Surg 2001;125: 265–9.

21. Videler W, van Drunen C, Reitsma J, et al. Nebulized bacitracin/colimycin: a treatment option in recalcitrant chronic rhinosinusitis with *Staphylococcus aureus*? A double-blind, randomized, placebo-controlled cross-over pilot study. Rhinology 2008;46:92–8.

22. Joe SA, Thambi R, Huang J. A systematic review of the use of intranasal steroids in the treatment of chronic rhinosinusitis. Otolaryngol Head Neck Surg 2008;139: 340–7.

23. Hissaria P, Smith W, Wormald PJ, et al. Short course of systemic corticosteroids in sinonasal polyposis: a double-blind, randomized, placebo-controlled trial with evaluation of outcome measures. J Allergy Clin Immunol 2006;118:128–33.

24. Weschta M, Rimek D, Formanek M, et al. Topical antifungal treatment of chronic rhinosinusitis with nasal polyps: a randomized, double-blind clinical trial. J Allergy Clin Immunol 2004;113:1122–8.

25. Ponikau JU, Sherris DA, Weaver A, et al. Treatment of chronic rhinosinusitis with intranasal amphotericin B: a randomized, placebo-controlled, double-blind pilot trial. J Allergy Clin Immunol 2005;115:125–31.

26. Ebbens FA, Scadding GK, Badia L, et al. Amphotericin B nasal lavages: not a solution for patients with chronic rhinosinusitis. J Allergy Clin Immunol 2006; 118:1149–56.

The Patient with Allergies

Christine B. Franzese, MD*, Neal W. Burkhalter, MD

KEYWORDS

• Allergy • Adult allergy • Atopy • Allergic rhinitis

Allergy is extremely common in the United States, with 20% to 25% of the general adult population affected by some form of chronic allergic respiratory disease.[1] Among children, allergic disease is more common, with some sources estimating that it affects up to 40% of children.[2] The social and economic burden of allergic disease is substantial, with allergic rhinitis alone responsible for 3.5 million missed days of work[3] and more than $6 billion spent on prescription medications alone for its treatment in 2000.[4] This does not take into account loss of productivity, physician office visits, over-the-counter medications, or other costs associated with additional manifestations of allergic disease.

Allergic diseases are ubiquitous in the United States, affecting all ages and walks of life, and they account for a large number of physician visits annually. Simplified, allergy is the undesirable clinical manifestation of an exaggerated immunologic response to an otherwise harmless antigen. These responses also are known as hypersensitivity reactions and are classified further into several different types, depending on the immunologic mechanism of the reaction. The focus of this article involves the manifestations of the most familiar and best understood of the hypersensitivity reactions, type 1 hypersensitivity, also termed immediate hypersensitivity. Type 1 hypersensitivity reactions are immunoglobulin (Ig)E-mediated, and the process of IgE production in response to exposure to an allergen is termed atopy. While type 1 hypersensitivity can be caused by ingestion of food antigens or pharmaceuticals, this article will focus on IgE-mediated allergic disease caused primarily by inhalant allergens.

Inhalant allergic disease may manifest in many organ symptoms. Allergic complaints, however, often are centered around the head and neck and upper airways, and because the myriad of symptoms all relate back to a single common pathogenesis, all allergic complaints frequently are gathered under the term allergic rhinitis. Much of the allergy literature centers around the diagnosis and management of allergic rhinitis, although the disease manifestations typically are not limited to the nose.

Department of Otolaryngology and Communicative Sciences, University of Mississippi Medical Center, 2500 North State Street, Jackson, MS 39216, USA
* Corresponding author.
E-mail address: cfranzese@umc.edu

Med Clin N Am 94 (2010) 891–902
doi:10.1016/j.mcna.2010.05.006
0025-7125/10/$ – see front matter. Published by Elsevier Inc.

medical.theclinics.com

Frequently, patients with allergic disease will state on initial presentation that they "have allergies." This self-diagnosis is often inaccurate. A patient's self-diagnosis should not be passively accepted without further query to establish the likelihood of allergy disease. Nonallergic triggers may cause symptoms that are identical to allergic rhinitis. These triggers include changes in the weather (or in temperature and humidity), air pollution, smoke, perfumes, fumes from household cleaning chemicals, or others. A patient with the previously mentioned triggers is more likely to have nonallergic rhinitis. However, it is just as common for patients to be completely unaware that the main cause of their symptomology is allergy. A good example is the patient with frequent sinus complaints who often feels ill from repeated infections. Many times, the cause is an underlying allergic pathology, not sinusitis.

An in-depth discussion of allergic disease and its many aspects of evaluation, diagnosis, and treatment is beyond the scope of this article. What follows is an overview of the most common manifestations of inhalant atopic disease in the head and neck, possible diagnostic options, and potential treatment choices.

HISTORY

For any patient with chronic or recurrent upper respiratory complaints, the diagnosis of inhalant allergic disease should be considered. The patient's history is the single most important source of information in making the diagnosis of atopy.[5] Additionally, there are various inflammatory conditions of the head and neck for which allergy may be a contributing factor to the underlying disease process. For some patients with head and neck symptoms, complete improvement may not occur unless the associated allergic issues also are addressed.

Sneezing, itchy or watery eyes, and clear rhinorrhea are common, well known allergic symptoms. However, other less specific symptoms also may indicate allergy such as complaints of nasal congestion, frequent sinus infections, change in hearing, ear pressure or pain, the feeling of ears being stopped up, or itchy throat. In addition, other disease processes, such as obstructive sleep apnea, eustachian tube dysfunction, asthma, and chronic rhinosinusitis can be exacerbated by inhalant allergies, so it is critical that the practitioner investigate the presence of allergic symptoms.

Timing and onset of symptoms are helpful to establish in diagnosing allergy. The onset of true inhalant allergies is rare in the infant and geriatric populations, but more common in the teen and young adult ages, peaking at around age 30.[5] However, a significant change in environment, such as a cross-country move, with exposure to new allergens, can be factor in the development of allergies in the adult population, so it is important to elicit this history when seeing a new patient with allergic-type symptoms. Whether the symptoms are present year-round or only during certain seasons is very helpful in diagnosing perennial versus seasonal allergic disease.

Family history and environmental exposures are also key historical information. Allergic disease is hereditary, and other family members usually will be affected by the same or similar complaints as the patient. The list of environmental exposures can be exhaustive when considering home, outdoor, and occupational environments, but key things to inquire about are the presence of pets (indoor or outdoor) or livestock, tobacco use, hobbies, stuffed animals, carpeting or draperies in the domicile, and type of heating or air conditioning, indications of mold or humidity, and nearby landscaping. Certainly it is impossible during one session to investigate all possible exposures, but if the allergic patient is not improving with appropriate treatment, it can be highly beneficial to review additional environmental exposures.

SIGNS AND SYMPTOMS
Ear

Otitis media with effusion is an inflammatory condition of the middle ear mucosa without evidence of infection. Otitis media with effusion is the accumulation of serous fluid in the middle ear space, which can be the result of or merely accompanied by eustachian tube dysfunction. The serous fluid in the middle ear space may cause a conductive hearing loss and a feeling of fullness of the ear, both of which are often the major otologic complaints in atopic diseases. Multiple authors[6-8] have established the relationship between IgE-mediated eosinophilic reactions and the presence of otitis media with effusion. Higher levels of IgE and eosinophil cation protein have been found in the middle ear of allergic children when compared with serum levels.[9] Although most of the literature linking otitis media to allergic diseases is in children, a strong pathophysiological link is well established and thought to carry over into adulthood.

Eustachian tube dysfunction is thought to contribute to the development of otitis media with effusion also. This epithelium-lined tube connects the middle ear space to the nasopharynx and is responsible for both drainage of and aeration of the middle ear space. The eustachian tube normally stays closed, but is transiently opened upon swallowing, yawning, sneezing, or crying by contraction of the tensor veli palatini muscle. This transiently opens the eustachian tube and equalizes pressure across the tympanic membrane.

Therefore, the eustachian tube is uniquely positioned to be a connecting source and cause of changes in the middle ear secondary to changes in the nasal cavity. It has been shown that patients with allergic rhinitis can develop eustachian tube obstruction after provocation tests.[10] It has been postulated that allergy may contribute to the development of otitis media with effusion in one or more of the following ways:

Middle ear mucosa as a target organ for IgE-mediated inflammation
Inflammation and edema of the eustachian tube leading to obstruction
Inflammation and edema of the nasopharynx and nasal cavity
Reflux or insufflation of infected nasopharyngeal secretions into the middle ear space.[11]

Eyes

Perhaps one of the most common presentations of allergic symptoms is that of rhino-conjunctivitis, or a combination of allergic nasal and ocular symptoms. The marriage of the two symptoms is quite astonishing; in studies of allergic rhinitis, more than 75% of patients had coexistent allergic conjunctivitis.[12] The eye is somewhat different than other target organs in that is has no mechanical barrier to prevent interaction with allergens. Conjunctivitis is sometimes largely thought of as a minor component of the allergic response, but 70% of seasonal allergy patients report that their ocular symptoms are at least as severe as their rhinitis symptoms.[13]

During the physical examination of a patient with suspected atopy, it is important to stress that in the examination of the allergic eye, close attention should be made not only to the ocular tissues themselves, but also to the surrounding periorbital skin.[14] In allergic conjunctivitis, the eyelids and eyelashes are notable for erythema, swelling, thickening, and discoloration (**Fig. 1**). The conjunctiva should be examined for hyperemia, scarring, and chemosis (clear swelling). The presence or absence of discharge from the eye should be noted, and any discharge should be documented with a description of its color, amount, location, and quality. Corneal injury is unlikely in

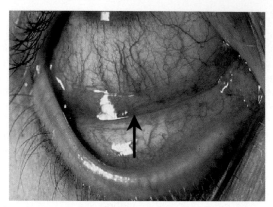

Fig. 1. Allergic conjunctivitis. Arrow indicates area of chemosis in the conjunctiva. (*From* Adkinson. Middleton's allergy: principles and practice. 7th edition. Philadelphia (PA): Mosby; 2008; with permission.)

acute forms of allergic conjunctivitis, but is common in more chronic forms of ocular allergy.

Perhaps one of the most striking ocular physical findings in the periorbital region of atopic patients has been termed allergic shiners.[5] The allergic shiner is a dark discoloration that appears below the lower eyelids, similar to how a black eye or traumatic shiner would appear (**Fig. 2**). This discoloration, which also can be hereditary, can present throughout any point in life, and if left untreated, the discoloration can become permanent. Another, more subtle ocular finding that frequently accompanies allergic shiners is Dennie-Morgan lines, or simply Dennie lines.[5] These are creases or folds the appear on the lower eyelids, underneath the lower eyelid margin (see **Fig. 2**). Both allergic shiners and Dennie lines occur from venous congestion in the orbital region as a result of nasal congestion. The venous congestion results in discoloration of the overlying skin, and it is hypothesized that localized hypoxia causes spasms of Muller muscle, which appear as Dennie lines. Leakage of hemosiderin can cause the allergic shiner discoloration to become permanent, with the possibility of Dennie lines becoming permanent also.

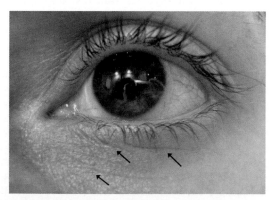

Fig. 2. Allergic shiner. Arrows indicate Dennie lines.

Should the general practitioner find these symptoms of ocular allergy, the standard treatment regimes are similar to other allergic diseases. However, it is highly recommended that one seek the expertise of an ophthalmologist if the patient does not improve quickly with routine treatment.[14]

Nose

Allergic rhinitis, commonly referred to as hay fever, is defined simply as an IgE-mediated inflammation of the mucous membranes of the nasal cavity. Although there is not a single etiologic or genetic factor, there are some predisposing factors. Multiple authors[15,16] have agreed that a family history of atopy, elevated serum IgE levels in childhood (before age 6), cigarette smoke exposure, indoor allergen exposure, and a higher socioeconomic status predispose one to allergic rhinitis. Additionally, there has been agreement that the risk of allergic rhinitis is lessened in the presence of a large family, involvement in a day care setting in childhood, infectious exposures during childhood, and the avoidance of antibiotics for childhood sicknesses.[15,16]

Allergic rhinitis can be categorized into two broad categories: seasonal allergic rhinitis and perennial allergic rhinitis according to the offending allergen. Seasonal allergens are pollens of trees, grasses, and weeds affecting patients living in more temperate climates. Because of their predictable pattern, these often can be controlled more easily with anticipatory treatment before the allergen season. Perennial allergic rhinitis typically is caused by molds, dust mites, cockroach allergens, and animal dander. As one might imagine, major sources of perennial allergic disease in the United States are dog and cat dander.

Classic manifestations of allergic rhinitis are sneezing, watery rhinorrhea, nasal itching, nasal congestion, and nasal obstruction.[17] While these are the most common symptoms, allergic rhinitis is often accompanied by atopic ocular disease, ear complaints, laryngeal complaints, and, perhaps the most serious, asthma.

Physical examination provides distinctive clues to the diagnosis of allergic rhinitis. Optimal examination occurs with a nasal speculum and an adequate light source. Often clear rhinorrhea can be easily appreciated as well as edematous, boggy nasal mucosa. The inferior turbinates can be classically seen as swollen, thereby blocking nasal airflow, and can be said to have a purplish or bluish hue.[15]

With excessive rhinorrhea, patients will have evidence of the allergic salute. Although this is more commonly seen in children, this physical examination finding can be appreciated in the adult population also. In dealing with their rhinorrhea, patients develop a characteristic maneuver of wiping their nose with the palm of their hand and displacing the nasal tip superiorly. Over time, this creates a horizontal crease just above the nasal tip.

Lower Airways

The diagnosis of lower airway hyper-responsiveness or even a definitive diagnosis of asthma has been linked to allergic diseases repeatedly. Several large cohort studies[18,19] have shown that the prevalence of atopic diseases early in life may be a heralding sign that they may follow a fairly predictable pattern from atopic dermatitis to allergic rhinitis to asthma, the so-called atopic march. It has been objectively shown that these phenomenon are intimately linked; nasal symptoms, nasal airflow and inflammation markers directly correlate with lower forced expiratory volume in the first second of expiration (FEV_1).[20]

Fortunately, it seems that allergic rhinitis and asthma have a therapeutic relationship also. Treatment of allergic rhinitis has been shown in a few studies to reduce the incidence and severity of asthma. There has been a concept of priming introduced in the literature, whereby a certain threshold of upper airway inflammation is reached and triggers lower airway changes during nasal challenge tests.[21] In fact, some have said that control of the upper airway is necessary to control the lower airway.[22]

Although there are disputes over the exact pathophysiology of the connections between atopic diseases, allergic rhinitis, and asthma, the coexistence cannot be denied. When considering the patient with allergic disease, lower airway hyper-responsiveness must be considered.

TREATMENT OPTIONS
Environmental Control

Although complete avoidance of all allergens is impossible, control and relative avoidance of known allergens may be effective and achievable. Patients who have seasonal allergies to pollens should be aware of their seasonal cycle and reduce outdoor activity during the pollen season (**Fig. 3**).

Indoor allergens are far more difficult to avoid. House dust mites, animal dander, and insect allergens are the major offending indoor allergens.[2] Main living areas such as bedrooms and living rooms should be free of carpet. If this is not possible and in those rooms with carpet remaining, frequent vacuuming with a double filtration system should be used. Air conditioning can often reduce humidity and can help curtail indoor mold growth, although infrequent changes of filters can promote mold growth and increase antigenic exposure. Mattresses and pillows should be enclosed in zippered, allergen-proof covers, and bed linens should be washed in hot water at least every 2 weeks and dried on a hot dry cycle.[23] Stuffed animals also can be placed in the drier on high heat weekly to reduce the burden of dust mite allergens. Perhaps the most difficult indoor allergen to control is animal dander; the only totally effective measure of control is to remove the pet from the home. Such a measure is often difficult for most patients to do. However, simply preventing the animal from entering the patient's bedroom can have a significant impact on symptoms from indoor pet allergens.

Antihistamines

Oral antihistamines are the most commonly used agents for the treatment of allergic rhinitis. Antihistamines have been shown[21,22] to control the symptoms of nasal itching, rhinorrhea, sneezing, and ocular irritation, but have not been shown to be as effective at relieving nasal congestion.

The major difference between first- and second-generation antihistamines is the ability of the first-generation, older agents to cross the blood–brain barrier (**Table 1**). This quality makes them well known for their sedative effects. This quality has been shown to have a significant impact on school and work performance.[2] Second-generation antihistamines have little to no sedation effect when compared with the first-generation medications. It is notable that cetirizine is a second-generation antihistamine and is considered less-sedating because of the variability of its mild sedative quality in patients.

Oral antihistamines are first-line therapy for mild-to-moderate allergic disease and specifically for allergic rhinitis. They are also very effective at alleviating ocular symptoms and are used commonly in combination with topical antihistamines.[24] Additionally, it has been shown that antihistamines may be used alone to treat allergic conjunctivitis but the addition of a topical vasoconstrictive agent is more effective than either agent alone.[25]

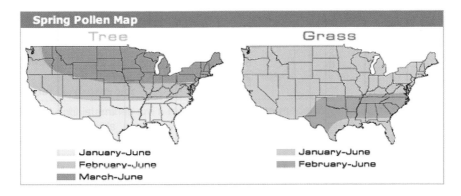

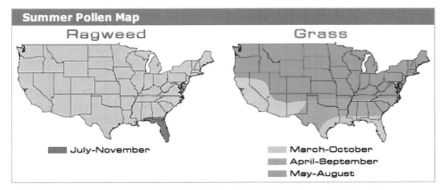

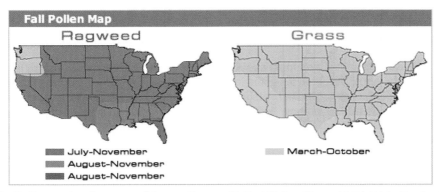

Fig. 3. Seasonal pollen map of the contiguous United States. (*From* AAOA Web site. Available at: http://www.aaoaf.org; with permission.)

Decongestants

Antihistamines are effective against a host of symptoms in allergic disease and allergic rhinitis. As previously mentioned, antihistamines have not been proven to be very effective against nasal congestion; therefore, combination therapy using an oral antihistamine and an oral decongestant has developed to target the full spectrum of symptoms. Decongestants such as pseudoephedrine and phenylephrine can be obtained over the counter. They are not without harmful effects, including insomnia, anorexia, and stimulation, causing difficulties with arrhythmias and exacerbation of

Immunotherapy is a very viable and effective option for some patients. Its effectiveness has been proven, especially for pollens and household allergens that are difficult to avoid.[29] Patient selection is critical, as there are some patients who are not suitable for immunotherapy. Patients taking beta antagonists or ace inhibitors are ineligible for immunotherapy given the difficulty in treating them for any possible anaphylaxis. It is appropriate in patients who:

Have failed adequate medical therapy or are having significant side effects from the prescribed regimen

Demonstrate IgE-mediated disease either through skin testing or in vitro testing

Will commit to a 3- to 5-year process of immunotherapy escalation and maintenance

Are controlled on medical therapy, but the regimen is too burdensome

Are younger with allergic rhinitis with concerns about possibility preventing progression to asthma.[5]

Additionally, some patients may desire allergy testing with or without immunotherapy simply to elucidate the offending allergens for the purpose of environmental control.

These and many other clinical situations are opportunities wherein a referral to an allergist likely would provide great benefit to the patient. The allergist would be able to provide further testing and offer immunotherapy based on the clinical symptomatology. Furthermore, one of the major advantages of immunotherapy is that it is systemic therapy and has been shown to improve symptoms across multiple organ systems.

SUMMARY

Allergic disease accounts for a large number of physician visits annually in this country and diminishes the quality of life and productivity of its sufferers. Allergic disease affects multiple systems through one common immunologic mechanism of IgE-mediated response, and its symptoms can range from annoying to life threatening. Predictable symptom patterns and physical examination findings will lead clinicians to the diagnosis of allergic disease. The treatment of allergic disease includes allergen avoidance, pharmacotherapy, and immunotherapy.

REFERENCES

1. Sibbald B, Rink E. Epidemiology of seasonal and perennial rhinitis: clinical presentation and medical history. Thorax 1991;46:895–905.
2. Dykewicz MS, Fineman S, Skoner DP, et al. Diagnosis and management of rhinitis: complete guidelines of the Joint Task Force on practice parameters in allergy, asthma, and immunology. Ann Allergy Asthma Immunol 1998;81: 478–518.
3. Kay GG. The effects of antihistamines on cognition and performance. J Allergy Clin Immunol 2000;105:S622–7.
4. Stempel DA, Woolf R. The cost of treating allergic rhinitis. Curr Allergy Asthma Rep 2002;2:223–30.
5. King HC, Mabry RL, Mabry CS, et al. Interaction with the patient. In: Allergy in ENT practice: the basic guide. 2nd edition. New York: Thieme Medical Publishers; 2005. p. 67–104.

6. Hurst DS, Venge P. The presence of eosinophil cationic protein in middle ear effusion. Otolaryngol Head Neck Surg 1993;108:711–22.
7. Tomonaga K, Kurono Y, Mogi G. The role of nasal allergy in otitis media with effusion: a clinical study. Acta Otolaryngol 1988;458:S41–7.
8. Bernstein JM. The role of IgE-mediated hypersensitivity in the development of otitis media with effusion. Otolaryngol Clin North Am 1992;25:197–211.
9. Bernstein J, Lee J, Conboy K, et al. Further observations on the role of IgE-mediated hypersensitivity in recurrent otitis media with effusion. Otolaryngol Head Neck Surg 1985;93:611–5.
10. Friedman RA, Doyle WJ, Casselbrant ML, et al. Immunologic-mediated eustachian tube obstruction: a double-blind crossover study. J Allergy Clin Immunol 1993;71:442.
11. Fireman P. Otitis media and eustachian tube dysfunction: connection to allergic rhinitis. J Allergy Clin Immunol 1997;99:S787–97.
12. Bousquet J, Knani J, Hejjaoui A, et al. Heterogeneity of atopy. I. Clinical and immunologic characteristics of patients allergic to cypress pollen. Allergy 1993; 48(3):183–8.
13. Wuthrich B, Brignoli M, Canevascini M, et al. Epidemiological survey in hay fever patients: symptom prevalence and severity and influence on patient management. Schweiz Med Wochenschr 1998;128(5):139–43.
14. Bielroy L. Allergic diseases of the eye. Med Clin North Am 2006;90:129–48.
15. Skoner DP. Allergic rhinitis: definition, epidemiology, pathophysiology, detection, and diagnosis. J Allergy Clin Immunol 2001;8:S2–8.
16. Ceuppens J. Western lifestyle, local defenses and the rising incidence of allergic rhinitis. Acta Otorhinolaryngol Belg 2000;54:391–5.
17. Rachelfsky GS. National guidelines needed to manage rhinitis and prevent complications. Ann Allergy Asthma Immunol 1999;82:296–305.
18. Gustafsson D, Sjoberg O, Foucard T. Development of allergies and asthma in infants and young children with atopic dermatitis: a prospective follow-up to 7 years of age. Allergy 2000;55:240–5.
19. Rhodes HL, Thomas P, Sporik R, et al. A birth cohort study of subjects at risk of atopy: twenty-two-year follow-up of wheeze and atopic status. Am J Respir Crit Care Med 2002;165:176–80.
20. Ciprandi G, Cirillo I, Vizzaccaro A, et al. Airway function and nasal inflammation in seasonal allergic rhinitis and asthma. Clin Exp Allergy 2004;34:891–6.
21. Spector SL. Overview of comorbid associations of allergic rhinitis. J Allergy Clin Immunol 1997;99:S773–80.
22. Corren J, Rachelefsky GS. Interrelationship between sinusitis and asthma. Immunol Allergy Clin North Am 1994;14:171–84.
23. Rosenwasser LJ. Treatment of allergic rhinitis. Am J Med 2002;113(9A):17S–24S.
24. Abelson MB, Paradis A, George MA, et al. Effects of vasocon-A in the allergen challenge model of acute allergic conjunctivitis. Arch Ophthalmol 1990;108:520–4.
25. van Cauwenberge P, Juniper EF. Comparison of the efficacy, safety, and quality of life provided by fexofenadine hydrochloride 120 mg, loratadine 10 mg, and placebo administered once daily for the treatment of seasonal allergic rhinitis. Clin Exp Allergy 2000;30:891–9.
26. Horak F, Stubner P, Zieglmayer R, et al. Controlled comparison of the efficacy and safety of cetirizine 10 mg o.d. and fexofenadine 120 mg o.d. in reducing symptoms of seasonal allergic rhinitis. Int Arch Allergy Immunol 2001;125:73–9.

27. Horak F, Stubner UP, Zieglmayer R, et al. Effect of desloratadine versus placebo on nasal airflow and subjective measures of nasal obstruction in subjects with grass pollen-induced allergic rhinitis in an allergen-exposure unit. J Allergy Clin Immunol 2002;109:956–61.
28. Bousquet J, van Cauwenberge P, Khaltaev N, et al, for the World Health Organization. Allergic rhinitis and its impact on asthma. J Allergy Clin Immunol 2001; 108:S147–336.
29. Nicklas R. Joint Task Force on practice parameters. Practice parameters for allergen immunotherapy. J Allergy Clin Immunol 1996;98:1001–11.

Evaluating and Managing the Patient with Nosebleeds

R. Peter Manes, MD

KEYWORDS

• Epistaxis • Packing • Cautery • Ligation

Epistaxis is a common clinical problem that is estimated to occur in 60% of people worldwide during their lifetime.[1] It accounts for approximately 1 in 200 emergency department visits in the United States.[2] Although epistaxis can occur at any age, the peak ages of incidence include patients younger than 18 and those older than 50. The episodes that occur in the older population tend to be more severe, whereas those in children are more often minor and self-limited.

NASAL VASCULAR ANATOMY

Epistaxis is described as either anterior or posterior. The origin of epistaxis has important consequences for subsequent treatment; therefore, a complete understanding of the vascular anatomy of the nasal cavity is helpful in defining both origin and treatment of epistaxis. Anteriorly, the terminal branches of the sphenopalatine and anterior ethmoidal arteries, and the superior labial branch of the facial artery, supply an arterial anastomotic triangle known as Kisselbach's plexus, located in Little's area (**Fig. 1**); 90% to 95% of episodes of epistaxis arise from the anterior nasal septum.[3] The external carotid artery supplies the internal maxillary artery, which, after dividing into multiple branches, terminates in the sphenopalatine artery, which enters the nasal cavity just posterior to the maxillary sinus through the lateral nasal wall. The two most common branches of the sphenopalatine artery are the nasopalatine artery, which supplies the posterior nasal septum, and a posterior superior branch, contributing to the middle and inferior turbinates.[4] The remaining 5% to 10% of epistaxis arise from these more posterior vessels. The internal carotid artery supplies the mucosa of the lateral nasal wall above the middle turbinates via the anterior and posterior ethmoidal arteries, which are branches of the ophthalmic artery. Epistaxis caused by anterior or posterior ethmoidal artery bleeding is quite rare, and typically only occurs in trauma with associated skull base fracture. These vessels may also be injured during endoscopic sinus surgery.

Department of Otolaryngology-Head and Neck Surgery, University of Texas Southwestern Medical Center, 5323 Harry Hines Boulevard, Dallas, TX 75390, USA
E-mail address: RPManes@yahoo.com

Med Clin N Am 94 (2010) 903–912
doi:10.1016/j.mcna.2010.05.005
0025-7125/10/$ – see front matter © 2010 Elsevier Inc. All rights reserved.

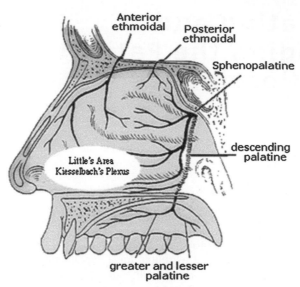

Fig. 1. Nasal septal vasculature. (*From* Viehweg TL, Roberson JB, Hudson JW. Epistaxis: diagnosis and treatment. J Oral Maxillofac Surg 2006;64:511–8; with permission.)

ETIOLOGY

The causes of epistaxis may be divided into local and systemic factors. Digital trauma is common, especially in the younger population. Mucosal dryness can cause episodes of epistaxis. Usually this results from low humidity or turbulent airflow secondary to septal deviations. Emergency room visits for epistaxis are reported to increase in the winter months, likely because of lower humidity during this time.[5] Chemical irritants may also lead to epistaxis. This may include both illicit nasal drug use and prescription topical nasal drugs, such as antihistamines or corticosteroids. Use of these commonly prescribed medications may result in epistaxis in 17% to 23% of patients using these products.[6] Patients should be instructed to direct the spray laterally, away from the septum, to decrease this occurrence. A simple way to achieve this is to have patients use their right hand to spray topical medicine into their left nasal cavity, and their left hand to spray medicine into their right nasal cavity. This decreases the likelihood that medication will be directed onto the nasal septum. Trauma can also lead to epistaxis. This is seen in the context of a nasal bone or septal fracture, and can be profound. Rhinosinusitis leads to increased inflammation and nose blowing, and may be a factor in episodes of epistaxis. One should consider the possibility of neoplasm as the inciting factor, especially if bleeding is persistent and no other cause is identified.

Systemic factors may also play a significant role in epistaxis. Hemophilia and von Willebrand's disease can lead to severe, difficult to control epistaxis. Thrombocytopenia, from either decreased platelet production or increased platelet breakdown, can lead to epistaxis. This includes, but is not limited to, hematologic malignancies, chemotherapy treatment, viral infections, and multiple autoimmune disorders. Chronic alcohol intake or renal failure can affect platelet function despite the presence of normal platelet counts.

Medication use can also contribute to epistaxis. Anticoagulants, such as coumadin, enoxaparin, and heparin all can be related to episodes of epistaxis. Nonsteroidal anti-inflammatory drugs (NSAIDs) affect platelet function and may contribute to epistaxis. Aspirin, which also induces platelet dysfunction, is implicated as a risk factor in epistaxis. A recent prospective cohort study of 591 episodes of epistaxis found those patients on aspirin to require more surgical interventions, to have a higher recurrence rate, and to have a larger number of required treatments.[7] Garlic, ginseng, and ginkgo all inhibit platelet function and can contribute to epistaxis.[4] A thorough medication history, including alternative therapies, should be obtained from patients experiencing epistaxis. For a list of medications that should be considered in patients with epistaxis, see **Box 1**.

The theory that hypertension contributes to epistaxis is controversial. Some studies have reported hypertension during episodes of epistaxis[8–10]; however, it is unclear if hypertension is the cause or the effect, as active bleeding may induce anxiety leading to an increase in blood pressure. Other studies have shown that blood pressures measured during episodes of epistaxis are comparable with routinely measured blood pressure.[11] Although there is no clear evidence supporting hypertension as a cause of epistaxis, it stands to reason that control of hypertension while managing epistaxis will not have a detrimental effect, and may aid in management.

Osler-Weber-Rendu (hereditary hemorrhagic telangiectasia [HHT]) is an autosomal dominant disease characterized by telangiectasias on the skin and mucosal surfaces. Epistaxis from HHT is often recurrent and can at times be life threatening.

EVALUATION

Evaluation of a patient with epistaxis should begin by ensuring a stable airway and hemodynamic stability. Once these have been established, a focused history, based on the etiologic factors mentioned previously, can help determine those contributing to the nosebleed. History should also focus on duration, laterality, frequency, and severity of the nosebleed. Although nosebleeds have the appearance of significant blood loss, most episodes of epistaxis are not life threatening. The presence of nasal obstruction, along with recurrent episodes of unilateral epistaxis, should raise the suspicion of neoplasm, which may be evaluated by physical examination and radiographic imaging. Trauma as an inciting factor should lead to an evaluation for other, associated injuries. Patients should also be asked about any family history of bleeding. Laboratory evaluation should be performed based on the history, physical

---

Box 1
Systemic medications associated with epistaxis

- Aspirin
- Warfarin
- Clopidogrel
- Ginseng
- Garlic
- *Gingko biloba*
- Heparin
- NSAIDs
- Ticlopidine
- Dipyridamole

examination, and amount of blood lost. This may include, but is not limited to, a complete blood count, coagulation studies, and evaluation of renal and hepatic function.

The physical examination seeks to determine the exact source of bleeding, but truly starts with a determination of the source as anterior or posterior. As stated previously, anterior epistaxis derives from the more anterior nasal vessels and encompasses the vast majority of epistaxis. Posterior epistaxis arises from the more posterior vessels and can be more difficult to visualize without the use of specialized equipment such as a nasal endoscope. Although the concept of anterior versus posterior epistaxis seems intuitive, it is of great importance, as the source of bleeding will help determine the appropriate therapy.

The physical examination should begin with anterior rhinoscopy, which allows visualization of Little's area, the source of many episodes of epistaxis. Suction, a light source, and a nasal speculum can aid in the examination of the anterior nasal cavity (**Fig. 2**). Topical sprays of anesthetics and vasoconstrictors, such as lidocaine or ponticaine with oxymetazoline or phenylephrine, can also assist in the examination. These can be administered separately or mixed together, and can be applied directly via spray or on cotton pledgets. Such medications can serve to slow the bleeding and make the patient more comfortable, allowing a detailed examination.

If no anterior source is identified, the bleeding is likely from one of the posterior vessels. Thorough examination of this area usually requires a nasal endoscope, as it can be difficult to visualize with the naked eye.

ANTERIOR EPISTAXIS TREATMENT

As many episodes of epistaxis are self-limited, patients will often present with a complaint of intermittent epistaxis in the absence of active bleeding at the time of evaluation. These patients should be instructed on a good nasal regimen to keep the nasal mucosa moist and prevent further episodes. Such a regimen may include nasal saline sprays, or the application of petroleum jelly to the anterior nasal cavity daily. Many other products, such as nasal saline gel, are available to serve as moisturizers of dry nasal mucosa. A humidifier in the home can increase the humidity of the environment. Patients should be counseled regarding digital trauma, especially parents of children with epistaxis.

When a patient does present with active epistaxis, many episodes will resolve with simple direct pressure. Patients should be instructed to pinch the anterior aspect of

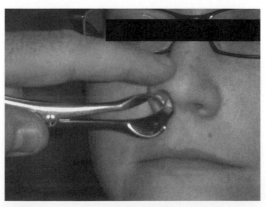

Fig. 2. Examination of the nasal cavity using a nasal speculum.

the nose for 15 minutes, with someone watching the time as a patient's perception of time will be altered, and 5 minutes of direct pressure will feel much longer. A common misconception among patients is to apply pressure along the nasal bones. This will not effectively compress the vasculature. Pressure should be applied at the nasal ala. Head position may be forward or backward, whichever the patient finds more comfortable, keeping in mind that a backward head position can lead to blood flowing along the nasal floor posteriorly, which may be aspirated or swallowed. This should be avoided, as further sequalae, such as vomiting or pneumonitis, may develop. Some advocate placing a cool washcloth on the face, the back of the neck, or along the upper lip. This will not cause any additional cessation of bleeding. Nor will pinching the upper lip or pressure above the nuchal lines. The primary method for stopping a nosebleed is direct pressure. Topical vasoconstrictors may also aid in cessation of epistaxis. These typically include 1% phenylephrine or 0.05% oxymetazoline. In one study, oxymetazoline spray stopped the bleeding in 65% of consecutive patients with epistaxis seen in an emergency room.[12]

If pressure and topical vasoconstrictors fail to stop the bleeding, cauterization can be used if a specific bleeding site is identified and accessible. Chemical cauterization uses silver nitrate, which can be applied to the nasal septum with minimal discomfort. The silver nitrate precipitates and is reduced to neutral silver metal. This reaction releases reactive oxygen species to coagulate tissue.[4] Brisk bleeds may fail chemical cauterization, as the rapid blood flow may wash away the silver nitrate before coagulation. A recent double-blind randomized controlled trial of epistaxis management in children compared silver nitrate cautery to sham cautery, and showed a small, but clinically significant improvement in the symptoms of the patients receiving cautery.[13] Circumferential cautery around the bleeding site before directly cauterizing the bleeding site is very effective at decreasing the blood supply to the offending area. Care must be taken not to prolong contact with the nasal septum, as perforations can occur. Also, only one side of the nasal septum should be cauterized at a time, again to reduce the risk of an iatrogenic septal perforation.[14] If bilateral cauterization is needed, the treatments should be separated by 4 to 6 weeks to allow mucosal healing and prevent the risk of perforation.[15]

Electrical cauterization using bipolar cautery can also be used, although this requires special instruments that are likely not available in all offices. The nasal septum should be anesthetized bilaterally using injected local anesthesia. Bilateral anesthesia is important because the electrical current can traverse the septum and significant discomfort may occur. Again, conservative, unilateral cauterization will decrease the risk of septal perforation.

Laser cauterization is often used for chronic epistaxis from hereditary hemorrhagic telangiectasia, with photocoagulation of the offending telangiectasias. Despite their effectiveness in this setting, lasers are not typically used in the management of acute epistaxis.

If the previously described methods fail to control the bleeding, the clinician should consider nasal packing as the next treatment option. Traditional packing consists of nonabsorable materials. Two common nonabsorable packs are a sponge composed of hydroxylated polyvinyl acetate that expands when wet (Merocel, Medtronic, Minneapolis, MN, USA) and an inflatable pack with a carboxymethylcellulose (CMCS) hydrocolloid coating that remains on the mucosa after the pack has been deflated and removed (Rapid Rhino, ArthroCare, Austin, TX, USA). Each of these packs comes in a variety of sizes that can be tailored to the specific patient, and some patients may require 2 packs per side. Longer packs can even provide some effect in the posterior nasal cavity. These packs are left in place from 1 to 5 days before removal. Failure to remove nonabsorbable packs, as can occur if a patient is lost to follow-up, can lead to infection or pressure necrosis of the nasal septum, especially when a patient has bilateral packing in place. In a randomized controlled trial comparing the previously mentioned 2 packs, both stopped bleeding in approximately 70% of cases that failed pressure and vasoconstrictors. In the same trial, however, physicians and patients found the Rapid Rhino easier to insert and remove.[16]

No matter which pack one chooses to use, care must be taken during the actual insertion. This can cause discomfort to the patient and, when done incorrectly, can cause significant discomfort. Also, placement and removal of packs causes some degree of mucosal trauma, which can lead to further bleeding; therefore, packs should be placed correctly on the first attempt. The pack should be lubricated with a topical antibiotic ointment such as bacitracin or mupirocin to assist in placement and for the antibacterial effect, which will be discussed further later in this article. A common misperception in placing a nasal pack is the thought that it should be placed with a superior trajectory. The pack should be placed along the nasal floor, which is parallel to the ground. Failure to direct the pack correctly will lead to unnecessary pain and trauma to intranasal structures. One should also ensure that the pack makes good contact with the mucosal surface thought to be the source of the bleeding. Failure to achieve this will result in continued epistaxis. The Merocel pack should be expanded using saline directly applied to the pack after placement. The Rapid Rhino is designed to be inflated with air via a syringe. The strings of the Merocel or the inflation device on the Rapid Rhino should be secured to the patient using tape, to keep track of what remains in the nasal cavity.

There also exists a variety of absorbable packing materials, obviating the need for packing removal later. These products include oxidized cellulose (Surgicel, Johnson & Johnson, New Brunswick, NJ, USA) and purified bovine collagen (Gelfoam, Pfizer, New York, NY, USA). These products act as a scaffold to improve clot formation, and can tamponade an area. They can be used separately, or together, by wrapping a piece of Surgicel around a piece of Gelfoam and placing it against the site of bleeding. Other products, such as porcine gelatin (Surgiflo, Johnson & Johnson, New Brunswick, NJ, USA) and bovine gelatin-human thrombin (FloSeal, Baxter, Deerfield, IL, USA) are mixed together to form a material the consistency of paste, which is applied with a syringe and is able to conform to the nasal cavity. However, because of their consistency, they do not provide much tamponade effect. In a study of 70 patients with anterior epistaxis, FloSeal was compared with a variety of different nonabsorbable packs, including Merocel sponges and Rapid Rhino. FloSeal was found to be significantly more effective at stopping nosebleeds, with a rebleeding rate at 1 week of 14% compared with 40% with other packs. Also, patients reported less discomfort with FloSeal and were spared the need for pack removal. Consumable costs were greater with FloSeal than packing, but this was partially offset by there being no need for a follow-up appointment for pack removal.[17]

POSTERIOR EPISTAXIS TREATMENT

If nasal bleeding is determined to be posterior in origin, there is limited role for digital pressure, medical management, silver nitrate cauterization, or standard packing. Although posterior epistaxis can be managed in consultation with other services, such as otolaryngology or interventional radiology, posterior packing can also be used and is quite effective. One case series reports a success rate of 70% in stopping posterior epistaxis using posterior packing.[18]

A traditional posterior pack involves securing a piece of gauze to a catheter passed through the nasal cavity to tamponade the offending site. Various balloon systems are available that also serve as a posterior pack. A double balloon device can be passed into the nostril until it reaches the nasopharynx (**Fig. 3**). The posterior balloon is then inflated, and the catheter extending out of the nostril is withdrawn so the posterior balloon seats in the posterior nasal cavity. Next, the anterior balloon is inflated to prevent retrograde movement of the posterior balloon. Again, an umbilical clamp is used to secure the balloon, with care taken to protect the nasal ala. If a double balloon device is not available, a 10- to 14-French Foley catheter may be used as well.

Overinflation of the posterior balloon or prolonged presence of pressure in the posterior nasal cavity can lead to serious complications, such as palate necrosis. The palate must be inspected after placement of a posterior pack to ensure adequate color, indicating appropriate blood flow. Furthermore, posterior packing should remain only for 48 to 96 hours. If using a balloon system or Foley catheter, the balloon may be let down but the pack left in place. This decreases the pressure on the palate, decreasing the risk of palate necrosis. But by leaving the pack in, one allows the physician to observe for rebleeding, and reinflate the ballon if necessary, without the need for completely new pack placement. If a patient has not experienced rebleeding 24 hours after deflating the balloon, the posterior pack may be removed.

Patients with a posterior pack should be hospitalized and monitored closely, as posterior packing may elicit the nasopulmonary reflex. The mechanism of this reflex is poorly understood; however, changes in arterial oxygen tension can lead to hypoxia and subsequent myocardial infarction or cerebrovascular accident.[19]

ANTIBIOTICS AND NASAL PACKING

When nasal packs are in place, topical antibiotics that coat the packs are often used, both to facilitate placement of the pack and to prevent toxic shock syndrome. Furthermore, patients with nasal packing in place are often on oral antibiotics directed against *Staphylococcus aureus*, again to prevent toxic shock syndrome. Coating the packs with topical therapy, although often recommended, lacks evidence that shows any

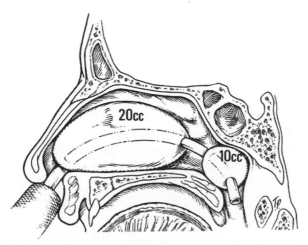

Fig. 3. Placement of a double balloon device. (*From* Cummings CW. Otolaryngology: head and neck surgery, 4th edition. Philadelphia: Mosby; 2005. p. 953. *Adapted from* Marks SC. Nasal and sinus surgery. Philadelphia: Saunders; 2000. p. 462. Figure 22–6; with permission.)

decrease in infectious complications. The incidence of toxic shock syndrome after placement of packing for epistaxis is unknown. A rate of 16.5 cases per 100,000 has been reported in patients who had nasal packs placed after undergoing nasal surgery, but the cause of toxic shock syndrome in this case is unclear, as it has been reported in patients who have undergone sinus surgery without the placement of nasal packs.[20,21] Despite a paucity of evidence, most clinicians will treat patient with antibiotics while nasal packs are in place, as the consequences of toxic shock syndrome can be life threatening.

COMPLICATIONS FROM PACKING

Complications from anterior and posterior packs include sinusitis, septal perforation, synechiae formation, and pressure necrosis of mucosa and cartilage. As mentioned previously, posterior packing can lead to nasal ala, columella, or palate necrosis. Although patients with anterior nasal packing can be sent home once the bleeding is controlled, they do require close follow-up, especially over the next several days.

TREATMENTS FOR PERSISTENT BLEEDING

At times, despite one's best efforts, none of the previously described methods are adequate to fully address epistaxis. At that point, consultation with appropriate services is necessary for definitive treatment. Further options include embolization or surgical intervention.

Embolization for epistaxis was first reported in 1974.[22] In this procedure, the appropriate artery is cannulated and contrast is injected to determine the source of bleeding. Once identified, the vessel is embolized with various materials. Common vessels embolized for epistaxis are the internal maxillary artery and the facial artery. Embolization of the ethmoidal arteries is rarely performed, as they are branches of the ophthalmic artery, and embolization may lead to blindness. Furthermore, the cannulation of the internal carotid artery increases the risk of stroke. Success rates for embolization have been reported from 79% to 96%[23]; however, complications include stroke, blindness, facial numbness, groin hematoma, and rebleeding. A series of 70 patients who underwent embolization for epistaxis reported one incidence of stroke. Thirteen percent of patients experienced a rebleed within 6 weeks of embolization, and another 15% rebled after longer follow-up.[24]

Another option for the treatment of intractable epistaxis is surgery. This may simply involve cauterization of the offending vessel, although if cauterization is all that is necessary, this can often be accomplished in the office by an otolaryngologist. Bleeding from the sphenopalatine artery can be managed by endoscopic sphenopalatine artery ligation. This can be performed in 30 to 60 minutes, and success rates are reported from 87% to 100%.[4]

Anterior epistaxis requiring surgical intervention is rare, but does occur. As stated before, embolization of the ethmoidal arteries is generally not performed. If surgical intervention to control anterior epistaxis is needed, an external ligation of the anterior and posterior ethmoid arteries is performed by an otolaryngologist. This involves a small incision near the medial eyebrow, with identification and cauterization of the vessels.

REFERRALS FOR EPISTAXIS

Although a discussion of surgical and embolization procedures is important for complete understanding of epistaxis management, most often these patients will have been referred to an otolaryngologist before requiring this level of treatment. In general, a patient with anterior epistaxis who has failed conservative measures, packing, and cauterization should be referred to an otolaryngologist. A patient with posterior epistaxis should also be evaluated by an otolaryngologist, with the understanding that, in the immediate setting, a posterior pack may be required to cease an acute bleeding episode. Typically, posterior packs are placed by an otolaryngologist, as improper placement can cause a significant amount of discomfort for the patient. But in an emergency, the previous description of posterior pack placement may be used as a guide.

If a patient continues to experience recurrent episodes of epistaxis, an otolaryngology referral should be placed. Recurrent epistaxis, especially unilateral, can be concerning for neoplasm and should be evaluated by imaging and direct nasal endoscopy. Other factors that may be associated with neoplasm include nasal obstruction, epiphora, or proptosis.

Last, patients with HHT should be referred to an otolaryngologist. Because of the potential seriousness of the epistaxis, and the understanding that these patients will likely need multiple interventions throughout their lives, having them establish a relationship with an otolaryngologist can assist them later in managing their disease.

POSTEPISTAXIS CARE

Once epistaxis has been successfully controlled, the physician must focus on treatment strategies to prevent recurrence. A similar strategy holds true for prevention of epistaxis in patients taking medications associated with nosebleeds, such as aspirin or warfarin. The use of nasal saline was mentioned previously as an excellent moisturizer of the nasal cavity. Many different topical gels and ointments are available to moisturize and promote healing of the nasal mucosa. Patients should be instructed in avoiding digital trauma, as this can often be a precipitating factor. In addition, patients should be instructed to refrain from nose blowing and strenuous activity for at least 1 week. Increasing the humidity of inspired air is also important. Patients may consider investing in a humidifier. Also, in hospitalized patients, oxygen delivery via nasal cannula should be avoided, as this can significantly dry the nasal mucosa. If oxygen delivery is needed, a high-humidity face tent will provide oxygen without the drying affect. If possible, patients should avoid irritants such as cigarette smoke or other chemicals that can irritate the nasal mucosa.

SUMMARY

Epistaxis is a common clinical occurrence, with a multitude of varying etiologies. Most epistaxis is anterior and will respond to pressure and topical vasoconstrictors. Cases that do not respond to these usually respond to cautery or packing. Rarely, surgical intervention or embolization is required for control.

REFERENCES

1. Viehweg TL, Roberson JB, Hudson JW. Epistaxis: diagnosis and treatment. J Oral Maxillofac Surg 2006;64:511–8.
2. Pallin DJ, Chng YM, McKay MP, et al. Epidemiology of epistaxis in US emergency departments, 1992 to 2001. Ann Emerg Med 2005;46:77–81.
3. Douglas R, Wormald PJ. Update on epistaxis. Curr Opin Otolaryngol Head Neck Surg 2007;15:180–3.
4. Gifford TO, Orlandi RR. Epistaxis. Otolaryngol Clin North Am 2008;41:525–36.

5. Walker TWM, Macfarlane TV, McGarry GW. The epidemiology and chronobiology of epistaxis: an investigation of Scottish hospital admissions 1995–2004. Clin Otolaryngol 2007;32:361–5.

6. Waddell AN, Patel SK, Toma AG, et al. Intranasal steroid sprays in the treatment of rhinitis: is one better than another? J Laryngol Otol 2003;117:843–5.

7. Soyka MB, Rufibach K, Huber A, et al. Is severe epistaxis associated with acetylsalicylic acid intake? Laryngoscope 2010;120:200–7.

8. Herkner H, Laggner AN, Mullner M, et al. Hypertension in patients presenting with epistaxis. Ann Emerg Med 2000;35:126–30.

9. Thong JF, Lo S, Houghton R, et al. A prospective comparative study to examine the effects of oral diazepam on blood pressure and anxiety levels in patients with acute epistaxis. J Laryngol Otol 2007;121:124–9.

10. Herkner H, Havel C, Mullner M, et al. Active epistaxis at ED presentation is associated with arterial hypertension. Am J Emerg Med 2002;20:92–5.

11. Knopfholz J, Lima-Junior E, Precoma-Neto D, et al. Association between epistaxis and hypertension: a one year follow-up after an index episode of nose bleeding in hypertensive patients. Int J Cardiol 2009;134:107–9.

12. Krempl GA, Noorily AD. Use of oxymetazoline in the management of epistaxis. Ann Otol Rhinol Laryngol 1995;104:704–6.

13. Calder N, Kang S, Fraser L, et al. A double-blind randomized controlled trial of management of recurrent nosebleeds in children. Otolaryngol Head Neck Surg 2009;140:670–4.

14. Schlosser RJ. Epistaxis. N Engl J Med 2009;360:784–9.

15. Hanif J, Tasca RA, Frosh A, et al. Silver nitrate: histological effects of cautery on epithelial surfaces with varying contact times. Clin Otolaryngol Allied Sci 2003;28:368–70.

16. Badran K, Malik TH, Belloso A, et al. Randomized controlled trial comparing Merocel and Rapid Rhinoin the management of anterior epistaxis. Clin Otolaryngol 2005;30:333–7.

17. Mathiasen RA, Cruz RM. Prospective, randomized, controlled clinical trial of a novel matrix hemostatic sealant in patients with acute anterior epistaxis. Laryngoscope 2005;115:899–902.

18. Viducich RA, Blanda MP, Gerson LW. Posterior epistaxis: clinical features and acute complications. Ann Emerg Med 1995;25:592–6.

19. Frazee TA, Hauser MS. Nonsurgical management of epistaxis. J Oral Maxillofac Surg 2000;58:419–24.

20. Jacobson JA, Kasworm EM. Toxic shock syndrome after nasal surgery: case reports and analysis of risk factors. Arch Otolaryngol Head Neck Surg 1986;112:329–32.

21. Younnis RT, Lazar RH. Delayed toxic shock syndrome after functional endonasal sinus surgery. Arch Otolaryngol Head Neck Surg 1996;122:83–5.

22. Sokolof J, Wickborn I, McDonald D, et al. Therapeutic percutaneous embolization in intractable epistaxis. Radiology 1974;111:285–7.

23. Smith TP. Embolization in the external carotid artery. J Vasc Interv Radiol 2006;17:1897–912.

24. Christensen NP, Smith DS, Barnwell SL, et al. Arterial embolization in the management of posterior epistaxis. Otolaryngol Head Neck Surg 2005;133:748–53.

The Patient with "Postnasal Drip"

Matthew W. Ryan, MD

KEYWORDS

- Post-nasal drip • Postnasal drip • Postnasal drainage
- Globus pharyngeus • Globus hystericus

Postnasal drip (PND) is a common clinical complaint. Patients use a variety of terms including "drainage" or "postnasal drainage" to describe their symptoms. In this article, postnasal drainage and PND are used synonymously. Although PND is a commonly recognized symptom among patients, there are rare citations in medical literature that address this symptom, the underlying pathophysiology, and the appropriate treatment. For example, a Google search for "post nasal drip" on 3/27/10 yielded 410,000 Web page results. However, a PubMed search on the same date, using the same term, yielded only 63 results in English, and a PubMed search using the compound term "postnasal drip" yielded 238 results. Most of this scientific literature is dedicated to PND syndrome as a cause of chronic cough and not to the symptom as perceived by patients. Thus, there is a profound mismatch between the attention that has been dedicated to the symptom of PND by the medical community and the lay public.

According to Sanu and Eccles,[1] who provide a fascinating history of medical accounts of PND, the first detailed description of PND in the medical literature was made by Dobell in 1866. Dobell described patients with abnormal sensations in the nasopharynx, mucus expectoration, and visible mucus behind the soft palate in the nasopharynx and oropharynx. The condition was referred to as "post-nasal catarrh." Dobell's description also included intermittent cough without overt pulmonary disease. A discussion of the causes and treatment of chronic cough is beyond the scope of this article, but it is worth noting that the role of actual postnasal drainage of sinonasal secretions as a cause of chronic cough has been called into question. The incidence of PND syndrome as a cause of chronic cough varies widely in the literature and may have a cultural basis, as evidenced by dramatic differences that have been found in studies from various countries.[2] Americans seem to be more familiar with the term postnasal drip and thus may be more likely to report the symptom to their physicians. Comparison of US and UK studies shows that the reported incidence of PND in patients with chronic cough ranges from 26% to 87% in US studies and

Department of Otolaryngology, University of Texas Southwestern Medical Center, 5323 Harry Hines Boulevard, Dallas, TX 75390-9035, USA

E-mail address: matthew.ryan@utsouthwestern.edu

Med Clin N Am 94 (2010) 913–921

doi:10.1016/j.mcna.2010.05.009

0025-7125/10/$ – see front matter © 2010 Elsevier Inc. All rights reserved.

from 6% to 34% in UK studies.[3] Other possible explanations of the clinical association of PND sensation and chronic cough, such as generalized inflammation of the unified airway and laryngopharyngeal reflux (LPR), are gaining greater recognition as the underlying factors that connect upper and lower airway symptoms. It has been argued that "'post-nasal drip syndrome' is a symptom masquerading as a syndrome,"[2] and perhaps because of the uncertainty, the currently recommended term for patients with cough and upper airway conditions is "upper airway cough syndrome."[4]

WHAT IS PND?

This is a useful question to ask the patient, as there is a limited vocabulary to describe symptoms. This vocabulary is derived from the local culture, family upbringing, and education. As shown by the author's Google search, the terms "postnasal drip" and "postnasal drainage" are quite familiar in our culture. Patients who present complaining of PND should be queried further to determine the meaning behind their complaint. Common associated terms for PND include drainage, phlegm in the throat, mucus, and cold. Patients may truly perceive mucus that is stagnant within the nose, and they may be able to sniff or snort this mucus back into their throat. On the other hand, there may only be a sensation that something is "stuck" in the back of the throat or a fullness in the nasopharynx. Patients may perceive a physical movement of something down the back of their throat but not be able to expectorate or remove any material. In addition, some patients use PND terms to describe the sensation of a lump in the throat, a need to swallow down something that they perceive to be in their throat, or the need to repeatedly clear the throat or the voice. The last description is more appropriately labeled a globus sensation.

Historical details that can contribute to a differential diagnosis include the onset, timing, duration, and severity of symptoms and aggravating and relieving factors. The most important historical data in these cases are the associated symptoms. In particular, the patient should be queried about associated rhinosinusitis symptoms, including, but not limited to, itchy, sneezy, runny nose; nasal congestion; nasal obstruction; anterior rhinorrhea; and decreased sense of smell. Detailed information about gastroesophageal reflux disease (GERD) symptoms and other throat symptoms such as hoarseness, cough, dysphagia, odynophagia, and choking spells should also be obtained. Benign-seeming PND symptoms may be the first manifestations of a nasopharyngeal, oropharyngeal, hypopharyngeal, or laryngeal malignancy, usually squamous cell carcinoma. Persistent or progressive symptoms, weight loss, and a concomitant neck mass suggest a pernicious process.

GLOBUS PHARYNGEUS

Globus pharyngeus is closely related to PND. Individuals may present for medical attention and complain of PND, when what they are really experiencing can be more accurately described as a lump in the throat, a tightness in the throat, or a sensation of the need to clear the throat. The symptom is usually most notable when making an "empty swallow," and individuals may swallow repetitively to try to clear the perceived lump in the throat. Up to half of the population may experience the globus sensation during some point in life, and during a 3-month reporting period in one study, as many as 6% of middle-aged women reported a persistent sensation of something stuck in the throat.[5] Symptoms may wax and wane over time, and spontaneous resolution is common.

Globus pharyngeus is referred to in the older medical literature as globus hystericus or pseudodysphagia, and indeed some studies have shown that anxiety can be a psychosomatic cause of this symptom. The symptom was described by Hippocrates as being more common in women and was felt to be related to the uterus. Because of its unclear cause, globus has long been assumed to be psychologically triggered.[6] The 1794 Oxford University Dictionary defined globus hystericus as "a choking sensation, as of a lump in the throat, to which hysteric persons are subject."[7] However, since at least the 1970s, the term globus hystericus has been supplanted by the term globus pharyngeus, and increasing attention has been paid to organic factors that may precipitate the symptom.

Globus symptoms usually include more than a simple feeling of a lump in the throat. PND and globus symptoms frequently overlap. The Glasgow Edinburgh Throat Scale (GETS) is an instrument to assess the spectrum and severity of globus symptoms. The GETS asks about symptoms such as feeling of something stuck in the throat, difficulty in swallowing food, sensation of the throat closing off, catarrh down the throat, and feelings of "want to swallow all the time" and "cannot empty throat when swallowing."[8] In a study using the GETS instrument to develop normative data on subjects who had not presented to an ear, nose, and throat (ENT) clinic for evaluation, the second most commonly reported symptom (55%) was catarrh down the throat.[5] Among patients with globus who have no identifiable anatomic pathology, 70% of subjects denied dysphagia or pain.[8] Globus and PND symptoms may be indicators of significant pathology, and atypical symptoms including persistent pain or solid bolus dysphagia should prompt further evaluation to define the cause.

THE PHYSIOLOGIC SUBSTRATE FOR PND AND GLOBUS SYMPTOMS

The PND sensation may be caused by excessive sinonasal mucous secretions, an increase in the viscosity of sinonasal secretions, or abnormal mucociliary function. However, The PND sensation is often present in the absence of actual postnasal drainage of sinonasal mucus. Furthermore, the PND sensation can be triggered by topically anesthetizing the nasopharynx. Thus the PND sensation is not specific. GERD is probably the most important organic factor that provokes globus symptoms[9] and is estimated to be present in 23% to 90% of globus patients.[10] Spasm of the cricopharyngeus muscle (upper esophageal sphincter) with or without extraesophageal (laryngopharyngeal) reflux may be another potential cause. GERD may cause direct irritation of the laryngopharyngeal mucosa, with direct contact of gastric acid with the upper airway. Other potential pathologic events include microaspiration of irritating stomach contents or esophageal irritation with vagally mediated effects and a vagovagal reflex. Esophageal motility disorders may also contribute to the patient's symptom complex. Other hypothetical causes for PND and globus symptoms include a large or elongated uvula, a curled epiglottis that impacts the tongue base or posterior pharyngeal wall, or an elongated styloid process with calcification of the stylohyoid ligament. In many respects, the pathophysiologic basis of PND and globus sensation remains unclear.

CLINICAL EVALUATION

The clinical evaluation of the patient with PND or globus symptoms relies primarily on the history and physical examination findings. Endoscopy, radiologic studies, and gastrointestinal evaluation are primarily performed to exclude significant pathology or to find corroborative evidence to support a particular cause. In practice, empiric therapy is probably the most cost-effective diagnostic approach.

The historical details obtained from the patient provide the most important clues to the possible underlying process. The spectrum of PND and globus symptoms may point to a sinonasal or reflux-related source of the symptom complaints. Patients often blame their symptoms on sinuses. However, an absence of typical rhinitis or sinusitis symptoms (other than PND) makes a sinonasal cause very unlikely. Patients with actual postnasal mucous drainage as the cause of their symptoms should have other accompanying symptoms such as anterior rhinorrhea, need to blow the nose, itchy or sneezy nose, nasal congestion or stuffiness, facial pressure or fullness, or nasal airway obstruction. PND that is secondary to a sinonasal source should worsen in tandem with other upper respiratory symptoms.

A reflux-mediated source of PND or globus symptoms is suggested by a lack of sinonasal symptoms and a notable relation of symptoms to eating or drinking, ingestion of certain foods, a full stomach, and so on. Typical GERD symptoms such as heartburn and regurgitation point to reflux as a possible cause. However, typical GERD symptoms are not uncommonly absent even though LPR is the cause of the patient's symptom complex.[11]

Other important historical items to ascertain include pain or throat burning, solid or liquid bolus dysphagia, pill dysphagia, food limitations, weight loss or gain, and tobacco and alcohol use. These historical items help to identify patients with possible malignancy, who should undergo further diagnostic evaluation.

Physical examination should include a detailed head and neck examination, with particular attention to the nasal cavity, pharynx, and neck. The nasal cavities may be examined with an otoscope to identify abnormal nasal secretions, mucosal edema and congestion, or nasal polyps. This examination can be facilitated by first spraying the nose with a decongestant nasal spray. Examination of the pharynx may reveal actual mucus draining from the nasopharynx into the oropharynx; usually this is identified laterally just behind the posterior tonsillar pillar. Oropharyngeal examination may also rule out pharyngeal masses or lesions. Without special equipment, it is not possible to examine the larynx and hypopharynx. Neck examination is important to exclude lymphadenopathy or thyromegaly, and some patients with globus symptoms have tenderness or soreness in the region of their larynx.

DIFFERENTIAL DIAGNOSIS OF PND/GLOBUS SYMPTOMS

The most commonly identified sources of PND/globus symptoms are sinonasal, laryngopharyngeal, or reflux related. Sinonasal inflammation that results from viral or bacterial infection, environmental irritants, or allergen exposure causes an increase in mucous secretion with changes in mucus viscosity. Simultaneously, the inflammation itself damages the ciliated respiratory epithelium. The combination of mucous changes and altered ciliary function leads to a stasis of secretions that may be perceived by the patient in the nasopharynx. Thus, conditions such as allergic and nonallergic rhinitis, viral upper respiratory infections, and acute and chronic sinusitis can commonly cause PND sensation. However, patients with these conditions rarely present with PND as their chief complaint.

PND is a common symptomatic complaint among subjects with chronic sinusitis. Orlandi and Terrell[12] evaluated the symptom profile of a cohort of 57 subjects with chronic rhinosinusitis (confirmed by computed tomographic [CT] scan) who were felt to be candidates for sinus surgery at a university medical center otolaryngology clinic. The most common symptoms (as reported from a standardized list presented to each patient) were nasal obstruction (80%) followed by facial congestion/fullness (70%), PND (67%), and fatigue (67%). However, it is also not uncommon for patients to blame their PND on a condition like chronic sinusitis. In a cohort of subjects who presented to a university otolaryngology clinic to be evaluated for chronic rhinosinusitis (CRS), 17% reported PND as their chief complaint and 61% reported PND as a symptom.[13] Not all of these subjects were eventually diagnosed with chronic sinusitis. For those with PND as the chief complaint, only 19% had objective evidence of sinusitis on nasal endoscopy. PND alone is not a specific symptom for rhinosinusitis.

Reflux is the next most important organic factor that provokes globus and PND symptoms. Indeed, research tools like the Reflux Symptom Index developed by Belafsky and colleagues[14] ask about symptoms such as excessive throat mucus or PND and globus sensation, as well as hoarseness, throat clearing, cough, choking spells, and typical GERD symptoms. Reflux can cause throat symptoms and cough without the typical GERD symptoms,[15] but even if these symptoms are present, patients do not often make a connection between their PND/globus symptoms and reflux problem.

The remaining causes of PND and globus sensation are rare, and the differential includes both benign and malignant processes. A variety of benign and malignant neoplasms anywhere from the nasopharynx to the esophageal inlet can cause these symptoms. Symptoms can be iatrogenic, as a result of pharyngeal surgery. Globus can be caused by thyroid masses or enlargement. In a prospective cohort study, a third of patients who underwent thyroid surgery had globus symptoms preoperatively and most improved after thyroid surgery.[16] An assortment of other conditions such as lingual tonsillar hypertrophy or cervical osteophytes may also be implicated after thorough evaluation. In a series of 194 barium pharyngoesophagographies, performed on adult patients (mean age, 51 years) with globus symptoms and no identifiable head and neck disease, the most common pathologic finding was cervical osteophytes, which were present in 32% of the patients.[17] Cervical osteophytes are common, however, and it is difficult to prove a cause-effect relationship between osteophytes and globus symptoms.[18] In many cases, no definitive cause of PND or globus symptoms can be identified.

MANAGEMENT APPROACH FOR THE PATIENT WITH PND SYMPTOMS

In patients with a suspected sinonasal or reflux-related cause for their symptoms, it is appropriate to institute medical therapy without further diagnostic testing. Often, the underlying cause is unclear, and patients may have overlapping symptomatic features that do not clearly point to a sinonasal or reflux-related cause. In such cases, an empiric treatment approach with close follow-up may be considered.

Treatment of GERD or LPR includes lifestyle modification and acid suppressive therapy for a period of at least 3 months. While clinical trial data are limited, it appears that LPR symptoms take longer to respond to medical treatment and do not respond to proton pump inhibitor (PPI) treatment as well as esophageal symptoms (eg, heartburn). For this reason, LPR is often treated with PPIs twice a day for an extended duration.[19] For example, in an open-label cohort intervention with daily PPI for subjects with GERD and LPR symptoms, 91% of subjects had significant improvement in esophageal symptoms versus 71% with improvement in globus, throat clearing, cough, or hoarseness.[20] Speech therapy has also been used by patients with globus, but its benefits are uncertain.[21] Reflux-related PND and globus symptoms may require months of treatment before benefits are recognized; patience with this prolonged treatment approach must be balanced with the imperative to diagnose serious pathologic findings early. Close follow-up of these patients is warranted until the clinical features or diagnostic workup has excluded a serious disease process. Fortunately, many globus symptoms resolve spontaneously.

The treatments used for rhinosinusitis as the cause of PND symptoms should be tailored to the patient's individual symptoms. Multiple medical treatment options that are already familiar to the internist are available, including oral and intranasal antihistamines, nasal steroids, mucolytics, and leukotriene modifiers. Any medication with a drying effect, such as oral decongestants or first-generation antihistamines, may be detrimental. If mucus viscosity or mucostasis are producing symptoms, it is rational to use intranasal saline to wash away or thin this mucus. High-volume saline irrigation is probably more effective for this purpose than simple sprays.

Clinical trials of medications for allergic or nonallergic chronic rhinitis have not been designed to specifically test the efficacy of these agents in alleviating postnasal drainage symptoms. For example, clinical trials for the treatment of allergic rhinitis typically calculate a total nasal symptom score that includes common symptoms such as nasal congestion, itching, sneezing, and runny nose but not PND. However, it is reasonable to speculate that if abnormal nasal secretions are caused by rhinitis or sinusitis, then medical treatments that are known to be effective for rhinitis or sinusitis will improve the symptoms. However, the effectiveness of common medications for rhinosinusitis is unclear. In one of the few studies to look directly at PND symptoms, Macedo and colleagues[3] performed an open-label study of medical treatment for 18 patients with a sensation of mucus in the throat and chronic cough (>8 weeks' duration). Patients with asthma and GERD were excluded. Subjects were treated with fluticasone, azelastine, and ipratropium nasal sprays for 4 weeks. The majority of these subjects had rhinitis or sinusitis as determined by nasal endoscopy and CT of the sinuses. There was no change in PND or mucus-in-the-throat symptom scores after treatment despite an improvement in anterior nasal discharge scores and nasal endoscopy scores. This study highlights the problem that effective therapy for rhinitis may not necessarily result in improvement in a patient's subjective symptoms of PND.

WARNING SIGNS OF SIGNIFICANT DISEASE

In some cases, patients with PND or globus symptoms harbor a serious pathologic process. However, a thorough diagnostic evaluation to pinpoint the underlying cause of PND/globus symptoms in every patient is impractical and expensive. The clinician must therefore rely on information from the history and physical examination to stratify patients according to their risk for a serious underlying condition. Symptoms that suggest a pernicious diagnosis include persistent hoarseness, dysphagia, weight loss, choking or aspiration, and a neck mass. The risk of serious pathology is raised in older patients with a history of tobacco or alcohol use and those with worsening symptoms despite treatment. A patient with these atypical features should undergo further evaluation to define the cause.

DIAGNOSTIC TESTING

There is no standard protocol for evaluating patients with PND or GERD. In patients without concerning symptoms, a trial of medical therapy is appropriate initially. A patient with a history that suggests the possibility of a neoplasm should undergo prompt evaluation with imaging and endoscopy. Otolaryngologists frequently use flexible laryngoscopy to rule out hypopharyngeal or laryngeal pathology and to evaluate for physical evidence of LPR, but this testing modality is not commonly used by generalist physicians. Other diagnostic tools can also be beneficially used in select circumstances.

The barium esophagram has been commonly used in the evaluation of patients with throat complaints. However, its utility as a screening test for all patients with globus symptoms has been called into question. Alaani and colleagues[22] reviewed the results of 1145 barium swallow reports for patients who presented with globus pharyngeus at Derbyshire Royal Hospital in England. Of these barium studies, 67% were normal. Abnormal findings were not uncommon but could be classified as benign: 18% showed hiatus hernia or GERD, 4% showed a Zenker diverticulum, 4% showed cricopharyngeal spasm or web, 4% showed cervical osteophytes, and 4% showed achalasia. In 12 cases (1%) there was a suspected tumor. Subsequent endoscopic evaluation and biopsy of these 12 suspicious cases failed to identify a tumor. This study and another with more than 2000 barium swallows for evaluation of globus[23] illustrate that barium swallow may be able to identify some contributory pathology, but cancer is sufficiently rare that barium swallow is not necessary for every patient with globus symptoms. Pain and dysphagia associated with globus are more highly associated with abnormal barium swallow results.[23] In addition, the sensitivity of barium swallow to detect hypopharyngeal or small upper digestive tract tumors is low. Therefore, barium swallow is not necessary unless patients have atypical symptoms (dysphagia, weight loss, pain) or risk factors for upper aerodigestive tract cancer.

Other imaging studies, such as ultrasonography, CT, or magnetic resonance imaging (MRI), may be helpful in selected circumstances to rule in or rule out various conditions that can cause PND and globus symptoms. In general, these imaging modalities are not as sensitive as endoscopy at identifying upper aerodigestive tract malignancy. However, a contrasted neck CT or MRI can evaluate suspected cervical adenopathy. The evaluation for suspected chronic sinusitis is greatly aided by a non-contrasted CT. A normal CT of the sinuses essentially excludes sinusitis but does not rule out rhinitis as a cause of the patient's symptoms. A thyroid ultrasonogram can characterize a suspected thyroid mass, and cervical CT or plain radiographs can evaluate osteophytes. Because many conditions like cervical osteophytes or a thyroid nodule may not actually be causing the patient's symptoms, imaging should primarily be directed toward the exclusion of serious treatable disease processes.

Twenty-four–hour pH probe monitoring has become the gold standard test for gastroesophageal reflux. However, because the test is invasive and uncomfortable, it is usually reserved for patients with refractory symptoms or in whom there is a need to be sure of the diagnosis. The nuance associated with pH probe monitoring and the diagnosis of GERD is beyond the scope of this article, but it is worth noting that the criteria for diagnosing LPR from pH probe data are unsettled. Dual probe, nasopharyngeal probe, and impedance monitoring are all used to capture reflux events that may be causing LPR symptoms. However, normative data for some testing approaches are lacking, and there is currently no gold standard to diagnose LPR.[19] Investigators continue to struggle with the correlation of throat symptoms, laryngoscopic findings, and reflux measurements in an effort to establish a reproducible diagnostic framework. This work will hopefully improve our understanding of the relative importance of various throat symptoms in making the diagnosis of LPR. For example, Smit and colleagues[10] performed 24-hour pH dual probe monitoring on a cohort of patients with globus symptoms, chronic hoarseness, or both. These individuals already had a normal flexible laryngoscopy examination. Pathologic reflux was detected in 72% of subjects with combined hoarseness and globus, but in only 35% of subjects with hoarseness alone and 30% of subjects with globus alone. Thus the combination of hoarseness and globus was more specific for the diagnosis of reflux. At present, pH probe monitoring should not be a routine part of the evaluation of patients with suspected GERD or LPR. These tests should probably be ordered by gastroenterologists and otolaryngologists in the evaluation of difficult cases with persistent symptoms.

INDICATIONS FOR REFERRAL

Patients with PND or globus symptoms that do not respond to treatment may have a condition other than reflux or sinonasal inflammatory disease that is causing their symptoms. If initial empiric medical management is not successful, a more thorough evaluation may be necessary. In particular, a thorough endoscopic evaluation of the upper aerodigestive tract is advisable to rule out serious pathology. For patients who present with signs or symptoms that suggest a serious condition, referral to an otolaryngologist is appropriate before instituting empiric therapy. Patients with weight loss, dysphagia, persistent pain, persistent hoarseness, or cervical lymphadenopathy have a greater likelihood of malignancy. In addition to sinonasal and upper aerodigestive tract endoscopy, the otolaryngologist may obtain imaging results or perform biopsies as indicated. The primary goal is to rule out a serious treatable process. After this has been accomplished, medical therapy can be revisited. In some cases, complete resolution of symptoms is not possible or no underlying cause for the patient's symptoms can be identified. In these instances, education and help with coping mechanisms can assist the patient in accommodating to their somatic sensations.

SUMMARY

PND is a common symptomatic complaint. In most cases, PND is part of a symptom complex associated with rhinosinusitis. However, gastroesophageal reflux is a common cause of PND complaints and should be distinguished from sinonasal causes via a thorough examination of the history. The treatment of PND is empiric and directed at the presumed underlying cause. Most patients can be treated without a thorough diagnostic evaluation. However, in patients who do not respond to treatment, or in whom there are concerning signs or symptoms that indicate the likelihood of malignancy, a prompt referral to an otolaryngologist for thorough diagnostic evaluation is advisable.

REFERENCES

1. Sanu A, Eccles R. Postnasal drip syndrome: two hundred years of controversy between UK and USA. Rhinology 2008;46:86–91.
2. Morice AH. Post-nasal drip syndrome—a symptom to be sniffed at? Pulm Pharmacol Ther 2004;17:343–5.
3. Macedo P, Saleh H, Torrego A, et al. Postnasal drip and chronic cough: an open interventional study. Respir Med 2009;103:1700–5.
4. Pratter MR. Chronic upper airway cough syndrome secondary to rhinosinus disease (previously referred to as postnasal drip syndrome): ACCP evidence-based clinical practice guidelines. Chest 2006;129:63S–71.
5. Ali KHM, Wilson JA. What is the severity of globus sensation in individuals who have never sought health care for it? J Laryngol Otol 2007;121:865–8.
6. Puhakka HJ, Kirveskari P. Globus hystericus: globus syndrome? J Laryngol Otol 1988;102:231–4.
7. Malcomson KG. Globus hystericus vel pharyngis. J Laryngol Otol 1968;82:219–30.
8. Deary IJ, Wilson JA, Harris MB, et al. Globus pharyngis: development of a symptom assessment scale. J Psychosom Res 1995;39:203–13.

9. Batch AJG. Globus pharyngeus (part II), discussion. J Laryngol Otol 1988;102: 227–30.
10. Smit SF, va Leeuwen JA, Mathus-Vliegen LM, et al. Gastropharyngeal and gastro-esophageal reflux in globus and hoarseness. Arch Otolaryngol Head Neck Surg 2000;126:827–30.
11. Koufman JA, Aviv JE, Casiano RR, et al. Laryngopharyngeal reflux: position statement of the Committee on Speech, Voice, and Swallowing Disorders of the American Academy of Otolaryngology–Head and Neck Surgery. Otolaryngol Head Neck Surg 2002;127:32–5.
12. Orlandi RR, Terrell JE. Analysis of the adult chronic rhinosinusitis working definition. Am J Rhinol 2002;16:7–10.
13. Rosbe KW, Jones KR. Usefulness of patient symptoms and nasal endoscopy in the diagnosis of chronic sinusitis. Am J Rhinol 1998;12:167–71.
14. Belafsky PC, Postma GN, Koufman JA. Validity and reliability of the reflux symptom index. J Voice 2002;16:274–7.
15. Irwin RS, Madison JM. Diagnosis and treatment of chronic cough due to gastro-esophageal reflux disease and postnasal drip syndrome. Pulm Pharmacol Ther 2002;15:261–6.
16. Burns P, Timon C. Thyroid pathology and the globus symptom: are they related? A two year prospective trial. J Laryngol Otol 2007;121:242–5.
17. Caylakli F, Yavuz H, Erkan AN, et al. Evaluation of patients with globus pharyngeus with barium swallow pharyngoesophagography. Laryngoscope 2006;116: 37–9.
18. Chen CL, Tsai CC, Chou ASB, et al. Utility of ambulatory pH monitoring and videofluoroscopy for the evaluation of patients with globus pharyngeus. Dysphagia 2007;22:16–9.
19. Ford CN. Evaluation and management of laryngopharyngeal reflux. JAMA 2005; 294:1534–40.
20. Oridate N, Takeda H, Asaka M, et al. Acid suppression therapy offers varied laryngopharyngeal and esophageal symptom relief in laryngopharyngeal reflux patients. Dig Dis Sci 2008;53:2033–8.
21. Millichap F, Lee M, Pring T. A lump in the throat: should speech and language therapists treat globus pharyngeus? Disabil Rehabil 2005;27(3):124–30.
22. Alaani A, Vengala S, Johnston MN. The role of barium swallow in the management of the globus pharyngeus. Eur Arch Otorhinolaryngol 2007;264:1095–7.
23. Hajioff D, Lowe D. The diagnostic value of barium swallow in globus syndrome. Int J Clin Pract 2004;58:86–9.

The Patient with Sore Throat

Teresa V. Chan, MD

KEYWORDS

• Sore throat • Pharyngitis • Tonsillitis • Laryngitis • URI

IMPACT

The National Health Care Survey in 2001 to 2002 reported more than 21 million outpatient and emergency room visits with complaints relating to the throat, and acute pharyngitis was diagnosed in nearly 12 million patients.[1] Although the underlying cause is often benign and the course is typically mild, the high annual incidence translates into a tremendous impact on public health from decreased productivity and overutilization of antibiotics. On the other hand, practitioners can make a significant public health contribution with small changes to their everyday practices. For instance, the addition of routine rapid streptococcal antigen testing on patients with presumptive pharyngitis reduced antibiotic prescriptions by nearly 50% in a pediatric emergency department.[2] Patient education and early identification of highly transmissible diseases, such as the 2009 H1N1 influenza virus, help to control the spread of disease and overall public health burden. Even seemingly basic symptomatic relief can speed the return to work and school and improve overall productivity.

ANATOMY

The throat anatomically consists of the pharynx and the larynx. It begins superiorly at the level of the skull base and nasopharynx, extending down to the esophageal inlet and most proximal aspect of the trachea. It is bounded anteriorly by the nasal cavity and oral cavity. The level of the choanae divides the nasal cavity and nasopharynx. A vertical line drawn between the junction of the hard and soft palate and the circumvallate papillae of the tongue divides the oral cavity and oropharynx. Disease processes limited to the oral cavity do not typically elicit a complaint of sore throat, and are not discussed in this article.

The larynx consists of the supraglottis, the glottis, and the subglottis. The supraglottis is made up of structures above the true vocal folds: epiglottis, arytenoids, aryepiglottic folds, false vocal folds, and ventricles (**Fig. 1**). The glottis extends from the

Disclosure: The author has no conflicts of interest to disclose.
Department of Otolaryngology-Head and Neck Surgery, University of Texas Southwestern Medical Center at Dallas, 5323 Harry Hines Boulevard, Dallas, TX 75390-9035, USA
E-mail address: Teresa.chan@utsouthwestern.edu

Med Clin N Am 94 (2010) 923–943
doi:10.1016/j.mcna.2010.06.001
0025-7125/10/$ – see front matter © 2010 Elsevier Inc. All rights reserved.

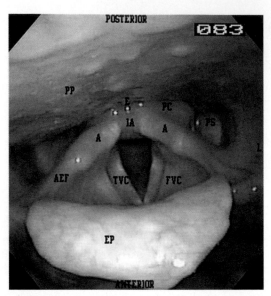

Fig. 1. Fiberoptic view of laryngeal anatomy. A, arytenoid; BOT, base of tongue; E, esophageal inlet; EP, epiglottis; FVC, false vocal cord; IA, interarytenoid mucosa; PC, postcricoid mucosa; PP, posterior pharyngeal wall; PS, pyriform sinus; TVC, true vocal cord.

horizontal apex of the ventricle down to 1 cm below the level of the true vocal folds. The subglottis begins 1 cm below the level of the true vocal folds.

The pharynx consists of the nasopharynx, the oropharynx, and the hypopharynx. The hypopharyngeal structures include the posterior pharyngeal wall, the pyriform sinuses that lie on either side of the esophageal inlet, and the postcricoid area that is the party wall between the larynx and the pharynx.

Sensory innervation to the throat is provided by the glossopharyngeal and vagus nerves. These nerves also supply sensation to the ear; hence, referred otalgia can be seen when the primary disease process involves the throat. Blood is supplied to this region by the ascending pharyngeal arteries and branches of the superior and inferior thyroid arteries.

CLINICAL HISTORY

Sore throat can be the presenting symptom of a myriad of different diagnoses. In most cases it is attributable to a benign viral process. A thorough clinical history will often help to differentiate these self-limited cases from those needing more investigation and possible referral to a specialist.

Because the complaint *sore throat* may mean irritation, scratchiness, burning sensation, or frank pain, the patient should be asked to elaborate on the description. In addition, from a patient's perspective, *throat* may refer to the entire pharynx and larynx, the soft tissues of the neck, or a single localized area. Having the patient indicate the epicenter of the discomfort with one finger can often be revealing. Discomfort that is located laterally and around the level of the hyoid corresponds to vallecular and tonsillar processes. Soreness or globus originating near the thyroid cartilage or cricothyroid membrane may indicate something in the hypopharynx. Globus at the level of the suprasternal notch could imply a foreign body anywhere in the esophagus. In general, well-localized symptoms are more concerning than diffuse complaints.

The duration of symptoms is an important indicator. Any sore throat that has persisted beyond 3 weeks deserves further investigation. Progression of the sore throat such as increasing pain or persistent irritation also warrants closer inspection.

The constellation of associated symptoms such as odynophagia, fever, voice change, and globus can narrow the differential and are now discussed in more detail.

Sore Throat and Odynophagia

Odynophagia or pain with swallowing is often associated with sore throat, particularly in infectious and inflammatory processes. Common clinical examples of sore throat and odynophagia include tonsillitis, peritonsillar abscess, thrush, and epiglottitis. It is sometimes the absence of odynophagia that is more helpful in narrowing down the differential. For instance, throat irritation from laryngeal reflux or postnasal drip will not typically be associated with odynophagia.

Sore Throat and Fever

Fever is sometimes present with infectious causes of sore throat such as tonsillitis, viral pharyngitis, retropharyngeal abscess, and epiglottitis. Exogenous pyrogens such as the lipopolysaccharides in bacterial cell walls or endogenous cytokines can trigger fever. Noninvasive fungal throat infections do not routinely cause fever; however, in an immunocompromised individual, the presence or absence of fever is a less reliable indicator. Fungal infections are notoriously opportunistic in an immuno-compromised situation, and must remain in the differential in these cases.

Sore Throat and Globus

Globus pharyngeus is a foreign body sensation in the throat. Patients will complain of "something stuck in my throat." Globus that can be well localized may stem from a neoplasm, a vocal cord granuloma, tonsilliths, or an actual foreign body. A more vague or diffuse sense of globus can also arise from edema of the postcricoid area (see **Fig. 1**). The postcricoid area is the party wall between the larynx and esophageal inlet, and can be affected by refluxed stomach contents from below, or infectious or allergic mediators found in nasal discharge from above. All patients with a chronic sore throat should be questioned about their allergic history and reflux symptoms such as prior diagnosis of gastroesophageal reflux or ulcer, epigastric burning, sour brash, chronic throat clearing, intermittent voice change, and globus.

Sore Throat and Voice Change

A peritonsillar abscess may cause a characteristic muffled quality to the voice, often referred to as a "hot potato" voice. This condition occurs because the soft palate is no longer able to move as freely due to tethering of the peritonsillar muscles and edema of the palate, which causes a transient velopharyngeal insufficiency and muffled oral resonance.[3] A similar voice change can be seen with significant hypertrophy of the tonsils from tonsillitis, or a disease process causing lymphoid hypertrophy such as mononucleosis or lymphoma.

The symptom of hoarseness indicates a process that has caused edema or irregularity of smooth free edge of the true vocal cords. Neoplasms or infections of the glottis can cause hoarseness directly. Neoplasms of the supraglottis or the hypopharynx can cause sore throat with hoarseness once the disease has extended to involve the true vocal folds, impinge on the recurrent laryngeal nerve, or involve the area between the thyroid cartilage and vocal folds called the paraglottic space. Moreover, progression of disease in these areas may lead to stridor or dyspnea, two signs that should always elicit an immediate airway evaluation by a specialist.

Sore Throat with Airway Compromise

A patient in airway distress may manifest some or all of the following signs: stridor, tachypnea, forward positioning with the neck extended to open up the airway, also known as "tripoding," drooling, cyanosis, or complete obstruction. These are signs that no practitioner should miss. Infectious, inflammatory, and neoplastic processes can lead to this picture. Common pathological conditions include epiglottitis or supra-glottitis, retropharyngeal abscess, parapharyngeal abscess or mass, and obstructing laryngeal and pharyngeal masses.

Sore Throat and Nasal Symptoms

Nasal symptoms such as congestion and rhinorrhea may be present with seasonal allergies or a viral pharyngitis. Nasal congestion or obstruction may also be associated with snoring and chronic mouth breathing during the day or night, which can cause a dry and irritated posterior pharyngeal mucosa and sore throat. It is also imperative to ask the patient presenting with sore throat about seasonal or perennial allergic symptoms such as nasal congestion, rhinorrhea, postnasal drip, palatal pruritus, itchy eyes, or sneezing. Chronic postnasal drip can also cause an irritated throat.

Sore Throat and Cough

Cough is a manifestation of airway irritation. Classification of the cough as wet or dry, productive or nonproductive, night-time only, or worse after meal times can aid in the diagnosis. A staccato "a-hem" or throat-clearing cough with a chronically irritated throat may be due to reflux or postnasal drip. Cough with an acute sore throat is more likely viral in nature. When cough is present with sore throat, it is less likely a streptococcal sore throat.[4] Cough can persist after resolution of the sore throat and other viral symptoms, and is thought to be caused by inflammatory irritation of the recurrent laryngeal nerve.

Sore Throat and Lymphadenopathy

Lymphadenopathy can occur with many reactive, infectious, and neoplastic processes. Notable posterior cervical lymphadenopathy is seen with infectious mono-nucleosis and mono-like illness. Anterior lymphadenopathy is present more often than other bacterial causes in streptococcal pharyngitis. Kawasaki disease is a pediatric autoimmune vasculitis that often presents with high fevers, lymphadenopathy, sore throat, and erythematous mucus membranes.

Timing

A sore throat related to extraesophageal reflux is typically worse after meals, when supine at night, or first thing in the morning. Similarly, postnasal drip related to allergic rhinitis can be worse at night or first thing in the morning. Chronic mouth breathing can lead to a dry and irritated posterior pharyngeal mucosa and a sore throat that is worse in the morning.

In summary, in patients presenting with sore throat the following elements their history should be sought: detailed description of the symptoms, specific location of the soreness, duration of symptoms, associated symptoms, timing of symptoms, presence of reflux, and allergic rhinitis symptoms. This evaluation will narrow the differential to a few possibilities and facilitate timely, appropriate treatment.

DIFFERENTIAL, WORKUP, AND TREATMENT

Table 1 outlines possible causes of sore throat. Some of the most common causes are discussed here in more detail.

Viral Pharyngitis

By far the most common cause of sore throat is viral infection. Common viruses include rhinovirus, coronavirus, adenovirus, parainfluenza virus, influenza virus, Coxsackievirus, herpes simplex virus, Epstein-Barr virus, cytomegalovirus (CMV), and human immunodeficiency virus (HIV).[4] The associated symptoms and season can give a clue as to which virus may be responsible. For instance, conjunctival involvement occurs with adnenovirus. The presence of ulcers may be due to Coxsackievirus or herpes virus. Profuse lymphadenopathy can be seen with Epstein-Barr virus, CMV, and HIV. Muscle aches would be more typical of influenza.

Viral pharyngitis typically is treated expectantly with fluids, antipyretics, and pain relief without further testing. Two exceptions to this are the influenza and Epstein-Barr viruses. These 2 viruses are now discussed in more detail.

Table 1
Common causes of sore throat

Class	Etiology
Infectious	Viral pharyngitis
	Influenza
	Mononucleosis
	Nonstreptococcal bacterial pharyngotonsillitis
	Streptococcal pharyngitis
	Peritonsillar abscess
	Tonsilliths
	Thrush
	Deep space neck infection (retropharyngeal/parapharyngeal space infection)
	Epiglottitis/supraglottitis
	Fungal Laryngitis
	Herpangina
	Syphilis
	Lemierre syndrome
	Fusospirochetal infection (Vincent angina)
Inflammatory	Laryngopharyngeal reflux (LPR)
	Allergic rhinitis with post nasal drip
	Chronic mouth breathing
	Foreign body
	Muscle tension dysphonia
	Vocal cord granuloma
	Mucositis
	Granulomatous diseases (rheumatoid arthritis, gout)
	Pemphigus
	Kawasaki disease
Neoplastic	Squamous cell carcinoma
	Lymphoma
	Sarcoma
	Adenocarcinoma

Mononucleosis

Epstein-Barr virus (EBV) is the causative agent in infective mononucleosis. Symptoms may include sore throat, high fever, extreme fatigue lasting 1 or more weeks, swollen tonsils with or without exudate, large anterior and posterior neck nodes, faint body rash, and petechiae along the palate. Lymphoid hypertrophy, in particular involvement of the posterior nodes, is one of the most distinguishing features from other causes of sore throat. Hepatomegaly and splenomegaly can also be present.

Patients who present with these symptoms should have a complete blood count (CBC) and monospot test. Because streptococcal pharyngitis presents very similarly, a rapid streptococcal antigen test is also warranted if there is any question. The CBC will show lymphocytosis with greater than 10% atypical lymphocytes.[5] Thrombocytopenia may also be present.

The monospot test is a serum test that detects the presence of heterophil antibodies with high specificity. The monospot does not detect presence of the virus. Heterophil antibodies are produced in the first 4 to 6 weeks after exposure. If testing is negative but the suspicion remains high, the test can be repeated in 1 week or antibody titers to viral components can be checked.[6] The combination of IgM and IgG to the viral capsid antigen, IgM to the early antigen, and antibody to a nuclear antigen (Epstein-Bar virus nuclear antigen) are helpful in interpreting the stage of infection. CMV can also cause a mono-like picture. IgM and IgG titers for CMV can also help to distinguish between primary, latent, or reactivated CMV infection.

The purpose of testing is to confirm the diagnosis and obviate the need for extensive workups for diffuse lymphadenopathy or fever of unknown origin. Treatment is supportive, with rest, fluids, and antipyretics. Antibiotics and antivirals have no role in the treatment of mononucleosis. Ampicillin specifically should be avoided in patients suspected of mononucleosis. If given, this will elicit a pruritic rash in most patients. Steroids are occasionally given for patients whose tonsil and adenoid hypertrophy has caused airway obstruction or sleep apnea. A nasal trumpet can also be used for sleep apnea related to adenotonsillar hypertrophy. Patients should be cautioned to avoid contact sports or other vigorous activity because there is a potentially increased risk of splenic rupture. The disease typically resolves in 1 to 4 weeks but may last up to 4 months.

If lymphadenopathy persists beyond this period, referral to an otolaryngologist for fine-needle aspiration, incisional biopsy, or excisional biopsy is warranted.

Influenza

Although influenza presents with sore throat, fever, and cough similar to the "common cold," it represents a unique global health risk. The virus spreads around the world in seasonal epidemics, and harbors the potential for pandemics such as the deadly 1918 Spanish Flu pandemic and the recent 2009 H1N1 pandemic. In comparison with other infectious agents, influenza virus has abundant natural reservoirs including humans, pigs, poultry, horses, and dogs. Influenza has a tendency to mutate, so vaccines must be revised yearly. It is spread easily via aerosolized droplets and direct contact, and is highly virulent due to frequent mutations. Strain to strain Influenza is also highly variable in its pathogenicity. Some viruses cause relatively minor symptoms whereas others are quick to cause severe disease and mortality.

Symptoms may include high fevers (>102°F/39°C), chills, myalgias, sore throat, coughing, malaise, rigors, and generalized body aches. Symptoms are typically more severe than those with a common cold. Physical examination findings are nonspecific.[7]

It is not cost-effective to test everyone suspected of having influenza. However, during an outbreak viral testing can help confirm those with the disease. These individuals should be counseled to avoid public spaces until afebrile for 24 hours. If identified in the first 48 hours of onset of symptoms, commencement of antiviral neuraminidase inhibitors may decrease severity of symptoms and shedding time of the virus.[8] Moreover, close contacts can also be started on therapy. This approach has been shown to provide postexposure prophylaxis against symptomatic influenza, although it does not necessarily prevent transmission of the virus.[9,10]

Annual influenza vaccinations are the mainstay of prevention. Vaccination not only protects the individual but also conveys herd immunity to those not immunized.[11] Its effectiveness, however, is contingent on how well the yearly vaccine represents the actual viral strain in the community. The vaccine is composed of components of influenza A and B, but science cannot always predict with 100% accuracy what strains will predominate. In these situations, antiviral therapy plays a more important role.

According to the 2009 Centers for Disease Control and Prevention guidelines, antiviral therapy with neuraminidase inhibitors such as zanamivir (Relenza) and oseltamivir (Tamiflu) are currently recommended within 48 hours of symptoms for all patients at high risk for severe courses or complications of influenza. This group includes the elderly older than 65 years, pregnant women, children younger than 2 years, and patients with certain comorbid medication conditions such as asthma, heart disease, and immunodeficiency. Patients with severe or progressive cases of influenza requiring hospitalization should also be started on antiviral therapy as soon as possible, preferably within 48 hours. Antivirals may be considered for all other patients. Treatment is commenced empirically, without laboratory confirmation of influenza.[12] Prophylaxis with neuraminidase inhibitors is recommended for the following patients who have had close contact of a person with suspected or confirmed influenza during the infectious period: persons at high risk for complications of influenza, health care workers and emergency medical personnel, and pregnant women. High-risk vaccinated patients who received vaccine in poor-match years and immunosuppressed patients who have been vaccinated are also good candidates for antiviral prophylaxis.[12]

Bacterial Pharyngitis and Tonsillitis

Several bacteria can cause pharyngitis and tonsillitis. Commonly involved bacteria include *Streptococcus*, *Corynebacterium diphtheriae*, *Neisseria gonorrhoeae*, *Chlamydia pneumoniae*, and *Mycoplasma pneumoniae*. Group A *Streptococcus* (GAS) is by far the most predominant causative organism. GAS is responsible for 15% to 30% of pediatric cases and 5% to 10% of adult cases.[4,13] Special attention is paid to identification of GAS because of the potential for preventable sequelae such as rheumatic fever, heart valve vegetations, and glomerulonephritis. *Streptococcus* is the only cause of pharyngitis for which antibiotics are definitely indicated.

Streptococcal infections are particularly prevalent in the winter and early spring. Patients with streptococcal throat infection present with sore throat, odynophagia, fevers, and anterior cervical lymphadenopathy. On examination, erythema of the tonsils and tonsillar pillars is present with exudates.

Several sets of clinical prediction rules have been proposed to aid in the clinical diagnosis of streptococcal pharyngitis. Two popular systems are the Walsh pharyngitis criteria and the Centor criteria. According to Walsh, patients who tested positive for GAS presented with a significantly higher frequency of recent exposure to streptococcal infection, presence of pharyngeal exudate, enlarged or tender cervical nodes, and high fever above 101°F/39°C. Presence of cough was a predictor of a negative

pebbles have the appearance and consistency of a kernel of cottage cheese. Tonsilliths are benign; however, patients are usually most bothered by the associated halitosis. Treatment of allergic rhinitis, pos-nasal drip, and extraesophageal reflux are reasonable initial measures. Active hydration with noncaffeinated beverages and gargling with nonalcoholic mouth rinses such as Biotene and Closys are also helpful initial recommendations. Curetting by the patient is not recommended because of the potential for bleeding. However, if the tonsilliths and halitosis persist, a patient may opt for a tonsillectomy, which is usually effective for both eradication of the tonsilliths and halitosis.

Peritonsillar Abscess

Peritonsillar abscess is a collection of pus between the lateral aspect of the tonsil and the pharyngeal constrictor muscles. A peritonsillar abscess is sometimes difficult to differentiate from a severe case of tonsillitis. Both present with sore throat, fever, odynophagia, tonsil hypertrophy, and possible tonsillar exudates. Drooling and asymmetric tonsils also may be present in both severe tonsillitis and peritonsillar abscess. Patients with peritonsillar abscess have a characteristic muffled "hot potato" voice, but the hallmark of a peritonsillar abscess, which is not present in simple tonsillitis, is trismus. Trismus indicates that the inflammation and pus has tracked above the tonsil in the pterygoid region. Pain that is worse on one side, asymmetric tonsils, and bulging of the palate are also tell-tale signs. A deviated uvula is not as reliable a sign in the absence of the aforementioned.

Treatment of a peritonsillar abscess includes hydration, incision and drainage, and antibiotics to cover common oral aerobes and anaerobes. A dose of intravenous steroids can help to relieve pain and trismus and allow access to the palate for drainage.

Needle drainage, conventional incision and drainage, and quinsy tonsillectomy have all been shown to have similar effectiveness in treating peritonsillar abscesses acutely.[23] Incision and drainage is preferred by the author when pus is found on needle aspiration. This is a procedure that most practitioners can quickly become competent to perform. One should keep in mind that the carotid lies 2 cm posterolateral to the tonsils and no that instrument should be placed deeper than 1 cm beyond the surface of the soft palate.

Common antibiotics used for peritonsillar abscesses include clindamycin, penicillin, penicillin and metronidazole combined, and cephalosporins. A culture typically is not obtained before commencing therapy, as it is not timely enough to dictate therapy and has no proven effect on outcome.[24] Antibiotic therapy should be aimed at covering both common aerobic and anaerobic organisms, as these abscesses tend to be polymicrobial. The most common anaerobic organisms found are *Prevotella*, *Porphyromonas*, *Fusobacterium*, and *Peptostreptococcus* species, whereas aerobic organisms are primarily GAS (*Streptococcus pyogenes*), *Staphylococcus aureus*, and *Haemophilus influenzae*.[25]

Peritonsillar abscess is a clinical diagnosis that usually requires no imaging. Ultrasound has been used increasingly by emergency room physicians for locating the pus when performing incision and drainage, with good reliability.[26] Radiographs will show soft tissue thickening and possibly the presence of air within soft tissue; however, radiographs are not the imaging modality of choice if one is needed. Computed tomography (CT) and ultrasound can be useful adjuncts when the picture is unclear or when the abscess is located inferiorly. An inferior pole abscess occurs only in rare cases but should not be missed, as it can more readily lead to serious complications including parapharyngeal abscess, airway obstruction, aspiration of pus with resultant pneumonia or lung abscess, internal jugular vein thrombophlebitis, carotid artery rupture, mediastinitis, and pericarditis.[27]

Recurrent peritonsillar abscess (>1/lifetime) is an indication for referral to an otolaryngologist for tonsillectomy. An interval tonsillectomy after the acute infection has subsided is often preferred over immediate (quinsy) tonsillectomy, except in the case of an inferior pole abscess when immediate tonsillectomy is the treatment of choice. Previous experience with quinsy tonsillectomy cautioned that higher rates of bleeding and other complications occur after immediate tonsillectomy, but recent reports have attempted to reverse this previous thinking.[28,29]

Parapharyngeal Abscess and Retropharyngeal Abscess

Retropharyngeal abscess and parapharyngeal abscess are 2 of the most common deep space neck infections, with similar presentations, workup, treatment, and concerns. A parapharyngeal abscess (PPA) usually arises from direct extension from pharyngeal and odontogenic infections. A retropharyngeal abscess (RPA) originates most commonly from retropharyngeal lymphadenitis. RPA may also occur after penetrating trauma to the posterior pharyngeal wall. Because the parapharyngeal space communicates with all of the other deep spaces of the neck, spread can also occur from one space to another.

A throat infection may precede presentation of the retropharyngeal abscess by 1 to 3 weeks, during which time these previously inflamed, infected nodes progress to central necrosis and suppuration. Retropharyngeal nodes are prominent up until 4 years of age when they begin to fibrose and regress. A typical presentation involves a young child, roughly 1 to 5 years old, who has had an antecedent upper airway infection and then develops neck stiffness, odynophagia, dysphagia, and high fevers. Any degree of airway obstruction may be present from a muffled voice to drooling, tripod positioning, tachypnea, stertor, stridor, and complete airway obstruction. There may be external neck swelling and the pharyngeal wall may be seen to bulge, though this may be subtle, especially if the examination is limited by trismus. Parapharyngeal abscess may present in the same way but tends to afflict an older demographic than RPA.

The retropharynx is a potential space that is bounded anteriorly by the buccopharyngeal fascia that surrounds the constrictor muscles, larynx, and trachea. It is bounded posteriorly by the alar fascia, which lies just anterior to the prevertebral fascia. The retropharyngeal space extends down to the level of the superior mediastinum around the level of the bifurcation of the trachea (**Fig. 2**). It is bounded laterally by the parapharyngeal spaces, which include the carotid sheaths. The potential for rapid progression to life-threatening complications exists on all sides.

The retropharyngeal space is separate from the so-called danger space. The danger space lies posterior to the retropharyngeal space between the alar fascia and the prevertebral fascia. It extends down to the diaphragm. The retropharyngeal space, danger space, and prevertebral space all lie in the same plane separated by millimeter-thick layers of fascia. Infections of the retropharyngeal space can be distinguished from the latter 2 by a midline raphe which, in theory, restricts abscesses of the retropharyngeal space from crossing the midline.

The parapharyngeal space is lateral to the superior pharyngeal constrictor and medial to the mandible. It is often described as an inverted pyramid with its base at the skull base and its tip at the level of the hyoid. This space connects to every other major fascial neck space and contains nerves, salivary glands, fat and, most importantly, the carotid sheaths, which extend to the mediastinum. If a deep neck infection such as RPA or PPA goes unrecognized, complications may include: airway compromise, rupture of the abscess with aspiration and pneumonia or lung abscess,

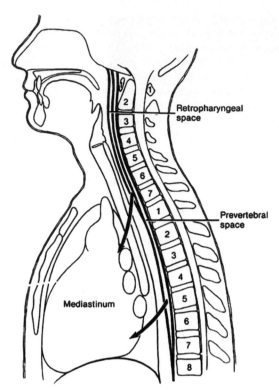

Fig. 2. Retropharyngeal and prevertebral spaces and their relationship to the spinal column and mediastinum. (*From* Flint PW. Cummings otolaryngology: head & neck surgery, 5th edition. St Louis (MO): Mosby Elsevier; 2010. Chapter 12, Fig. 12–20; with permission.)

extension to parapharyngeal spaces, internal jugular vein thrombosis, vertebral osteomyelitis, vertebral body subluxation, spinal abscesses, mediastinitis, pericarditis, and sepsis.

Workup includes first and foremost, airway management. If a patient presents with a suspected deep neck abscess, a plan for airway management needs to be determined from the start. Even those patients who are seemingly stable can be tipped over to a life-threatening emergency by thoughtless airway manipulation. Airway management options include observation with continuous monitoring, fiberoptic or direct intubation, tracheostomy, and cricothyroidotomy. Minimal palpation of the abscess, limiting oropharyngeal instrumentation, and avoidance of sedation are recommended when outside of a controlled and prepared environment such as an operating room. Airway management should ideally be done by the physician(s) who will provide definitive therapy. An otolaryngology consultation should be initiated immediately for laryngoscopic assessment of the entire airway, and anesthetists should be made aware of impending airway needs.

Once the patient is deemed stable, a workup can be initiated. Neck radiographs are a quick method of assessment and do not require the patient to lay supine. Radiography is a good initial study that can quickly help to triage a patient in the proper direction of care. A lateral neck radiograph in the setting of retropharyngeal abscess may show soft tissue thickening or free air in the posterior pharyngeal soft tissues (**Fig. 3**). A good rule of thumb is that if the width of the overlying soft tissues is greater

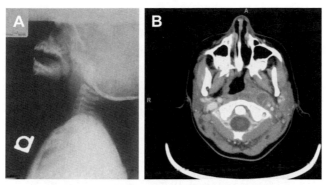

Fig. 3. Retropharyngeal abscess. (*A*) lateral neck radiograph shows widening of the soft tissues anterior to the vertebral bodies. (*From* Flint PW. Cummings otolaryngology: head & neck surgery, 5th edition. St. Louis (MO): Mosby Elsevier; 2010. Chapter 196, Fig. 196-7A and B; with permission.) (*B*) CT scan with contrast of neck shows rim-enhancing collection consistent with a left retropharyngeal abscess. (*Courtesy of* Guy Efune, MD, Dallas, TX.)

than one-half the width of the corresponding vertebrae, there is significant swelling that should be evaluated further. This method is gross but easily applied. Any radiograph, however, is greatly limited if the patient's neck is not fully extended and the film is not taken during end-inspiration. These suboptimal positions may yield a false-positive result. Lateral neck films were found to have a sensitivity of 83% for determining the presence of a pediatric deep neck infection, whereas CT scanning with contrast had a sensitivity of 100%.[30]

CT of the neck with contrast remains the study of choice for evaluation of suspected deep space neck infection (see **Fig. 3; Fig. 4**). From a respiratory and hemodynamic standpoint the patient must be stable enough to travel to radiology. Excessive secretions may preclude lying supine for the entire scan. CT findings include a rim-enhanced area of low density, loss of fat stranding, edema of the surrounding tissues, and possible deviation of nearby structures such as the airway. With RPA there is some controversy as to what specific radiographic findings are consistent with pus at the time of incision and drainage.[31–33] Some investigators advocate that irregularity of the abscess wall was a stronger predictor than just rim enhancement for the presence of pus at the time of incision and drainage.[33]

Although the information from a magnetic resonance (MR) image may be superior to that of CT for evaluation of deep space neck infections, the longer duration lying supine and the remote location are undesirable. MR imaging is also often not tolerated by young children without sedation. The ultrasound does not provide the spatial relationships necessary to assist in localizing the collection intraoperatively.

CBC and blood cultures should be checked and broad-spectrum antibiotics commenced without delay. Antibiotics should be directed at a polymicrobial mix of gram-positive aerobes and anaerobic organisms. GAS, *S aureus*, and *H influenzae* are common aerobic organisms that are found. Anaerobes include *Eikenella* (formerly *Bacteroides*), *Peptostreptococcus*, *Fusobacterium*, and *Prevotella*.[25] Clindamycin is the usual antibiotic of choice, as it has both gram-positive and anaerobic coverage. A β-lactam resistant cephalosporin may be used in combination with clindamycin. β-Lactamase has been found to be present in up to 60% to 70% of organisms.[34,35]

Parapharyngeal abscesses are drained immediately. The potential for tracheostomy at the time of surgery should always be considered and discussed in the consent. The approach to treatment of retropharyngeal abscesses is changing. Studies have shown

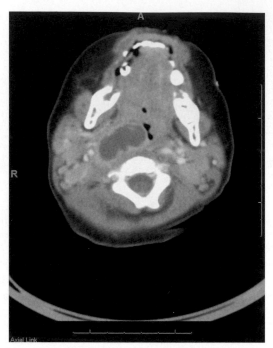

Fig. 4. Right parapharyngeal abscess with impingement on the airway. (*Courtesy of* Tim Booth, MD, Department of Radiology, Children's Medical Center, Dallas, TX.)

that a trial of intravenous antibiotics for small (<2 cm), limited retropharyngeal abscesses is often effective and may obviate the need for surgery.[36,37] Failure to improve after 48 hours of antibiotics is an indication for incision and drainage. If incision and drainage is performed, a culture should be obtained to help direct therapy. Unusual organisms such as m. tuberculosis should be suspected in patients who are refractory to conventional therapies or who have traveled outside the United States.

Supraglottitis/Epiglottis

Supraglottitis is an inflammation of any of the supraglottic structures including the epiglottis, arytenoids, aryepiglottic folds, and false vocal folds. It is usually of an infectious origin and more is commonly referred to as epiglottitis because of the prominent cherry-red epiglottis seen in affected children.

Epiglottitis was formerly an affliction of toddlers and young children aged 2 to 7 years. However, since the widespread use of the *Haemophilus* type B vaccine starting in 1985, the incidence of pediatric epiglottitis in countries that mandate vaccination has decreased dramatically.[38] Despite this decline, there have been documented cases of *Haemophilus* type B positive cultures from previously immunized patients with epiglottitis.[39] The incidence of adult supraglottitis in the meantime has remained stable, and may be increasing.[39,40]

Patients present with history of sore throat, high fevers, and odynophagia so severe that the patient refuses to eat or drink. On examination the patient often appears acutely ill and may have any degree of airway involvement including muffled voice, inspiratory stridor, tachypnea, drooling, tripod positioning, and use of accessory muscles. The patient may have an exquisitely tender anterior neck.

When epiglottitis is suspected, management of the airway is paramount. This disease process can progress rapidly to airway compromise within hours. Otolaryngology and anesthesiology consultations should be initiated immediately. In pediatric patients, any intervention including placement of intravenous access, imaging studies, and invasive examinations such as laryngoscopy should be avoided. Although the typical cherry-red epiglottis can sometimes be seen on oral examination, great caution should be used with any potentially stimulating examination. The child must be kept calm and comfortable. Sedatives and narcotics should be used very sparingly. The patient's airway is ideally assessed in the operating room with readiness for definitive airway management including nasotracheal intubation, oral intubation, or tracheostomy. A CBC, surface cultures, and blood cultures can be obtained at this time. If time will not allow and the patient's airway needs to be secured emergently, a cricothyroidotomy should be performed immediately, followed by endoscopy in the operating room, and revision of the cricothyroidotomy site to a tracheostomy.

The approach to the adult and adolescent patient with supraglottitis differs slightly. Older patients tend to be able to tolerate laryngoscopy and are more often managed with close observation in the intensive care unit with or without intubation.

Laryngoscopy is more sensitive than radiography in making the diagnosis, and provides a quicker definitive diagnosis than CT. If a radiograph is obtained, a widened epiglottis on lateral neck radiograph, referred to as the thumb sign, is a classic finding (**Fig. 5**). If associated abscess is suspected, a CT scan is warranted after the airway has been assessed and secured.

Whereas *Haemophilus* type B predominated in the past, nowadays *S aureus* and *Streptococcus* species are more often seen.[39] Clindamycin, cephalosporins, and β-lactamase resistant penicillins are typical first-line antibiotics. Intravenous steroids are also frequently given, although no there are no studies to prove their efficacy in

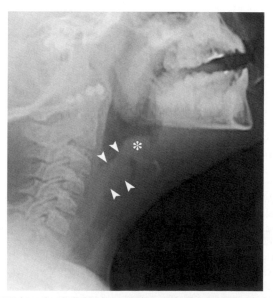

Fig. 5. Epiglottitis. Widened epiglottis (*asterisk*) and aryepiglottic folds (*arrowheads*). (*From* Flint PW. Cummings otolaryngology: head & neck surgery, 5th edition. St Louis (MO): Mosby Elsevier; 2010. Chapter 102, Fig. 102–30; with permission.)

resolving the disease process more quickly. Racemic epinephrine, frequently used in other airway emergencies, provides no improvement in epiglottitis.

Opportunistic fungal infections occasionally can cause a supraglottis that is more insidious in onset. Chronic throat irritation and voice change are common presenting symptoms. Immunosuppression or regular use of an inhaled particulate steroid such as fluticasone/salmetrol diskus (Advair) in immunocompetent patients can predispose to fungal supraglottitis. *Candida* is the most commonly involved fungus but in endemic areas *Coccidioides*, *Histoplasma*, *Cryptococcus*, and *Blastomyces* may also be present. Fungal supraglottitis is treated with systemic antifungals and by addressing the underlying etiology.

Laryngopharyngeal Reflux

Gastroesophageal reflux (GER) and laryngopharyngeal reflux (LPR) are increasingly implicated in diseases of the upper aerodigestive tract. Since the 1990s reflux has been considered a contributor to laryngeal irritation, and more recently studies have sought to understand its role in chronic nonspecific pharyngitis.[41] The mucosa of the larynx and pharynx are more sensitive to acid and pepsin than the gastric or esophageal mucosa. The larynx and pharynx lack bicarbonate production and peristalsis, which are protective to the stomach and esophagus. Koufman[42] demonstrated that even trace amounts of reflux, 3 times a week, are enough to cause mucosa trauma to the larynx. Recent studies in cell culture have shown that pepsin can damage hypopharyngeal cells in the absence of acid.[43]

LPR is thought to be a distinct entity from GER. GER is a high-volume problem whereas LPR is a low-volume, high-susceptibility problem. Those with LPR are typically daytime upright refluxers whereas patients with GER are symptomatically worse when supine. Symptoms of LPR can be present in the absence of common gastroesophageal reflux symptoms such as sour brash and heartburn. Only about 25% of patients with LPR develop esophagitis. Some patients may suffer from both problems and have a mixture of associated symptoms.

Patients with nonspecific pharyngitis may complain of a chronically irritated or sore throat, globus sensation, and chronic throat clearing. Intermittent hoarseness may also be present. Symptoms are typically worse after a meal or possibly after lying supine. Sore throat may be the result of direct irritation or chronic coughing.

Studies have shown that patients with complaint of chronic sore throat for which no other attributable cause was found scored higher on both reflux symptoms and reflux findings. Their symptom and finding scores also decreased compared with controls after 2 months of twice-daily proton pump inhibitor (PPI) therapy.[41]

There are 3 approaches to confirming the diagnosis of LPR: (1) response of symptoms to behavioral and empiric medical treatment, (2) endoscopic observation of mucosal injury, and (3) demonstration of reflux events by impedance and pH-monitoring studies or barium swallow esophagram. The first approach can be trialed by any primary practitioner. The latter 2 require referral to either an otolaryngologist or gastroenterologist for evaluation. On laryngoscopic examination, patients may manifest edema of the posterior glottis including the arytenoids and interarytenoid area. Erythema may also be present along the posterior glottis and posterior pharyngeal wall. There may be hypervascularity or edema of the true vocal folds (**Fig. 6**).

Behavioral modifications PPIs such as omeprazole, rabeprazole, esomeprazole, lansoprazole, and pantoprazole are the treatments of choice for LPR. Treatment can be initially commenced on the basis of laryngoscopic findings alone. Behavioral modifications include eating smaller and more frequent meals, not lying supine after a meal, avoiding a pre-bedtime or midnight snack, and raising the head of bed 6 to

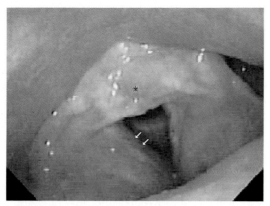

Fig. 6. Laryngeal changes from chronic reflux. Edema of the interarytenoid mucosa (*asterisk*). Irregular, edematous, and erythematous true vocal cord mucosa (*arrowheads*). (*Courtesy of* Ted Mau, MD, PhD, Dallas, TX.)

8 inches by placing on cinderblocks or phone books under the uppermost bedposts. Patients should also be given a list of reflux-provoking foods to avoid such as caffeine, mints, chocolate, tomato sauces, fried or fatty foods, high-cholesterol foods, spicy foods, carbonated beverages, and citrus.

There are 2 theories of drug therapy: a "step-up" method and a "step-down" method. In the step-up method, patients are started first on antacids, advanced to H2 blockers if still symptomatic, then started on daily PPIs, and finally twice-daily therapy if this is not effective. Alternatively, some advocate that starting on twice-daily therapy and then stepping down is more effective and less costly in the long run.[44] Patients should be counseled that it is important to take the PPI 30 minutes before meals for optimal effect. Two to 3 months of therapy usually are required to see effects. Persistent symptoms despite compliant therapy warrant referral to a specialist for further evaluation and consideration of surgical intervention such as a fundoplication.

Rhinitis

Rhinitis or rhinosinusitis may be caused by allergic, infectious, or inflammatory diseases. Patients may present with nasal congestion, rhinorrhea, postnasal drip, or nasal irritation. Nasal congestion, nasal obstruction, and postnasal drip can all contribute to a chronically sore throat.

Postnasal drip itself is not a pathological phenomenon. It is the conscious sensation of a naturally occurring process caused by increased volume or increased viscosity of the mucus. Mucus is secreted by the nasal mucosa with the purpose of trapping irritants, pollutants, infectious organisms, and allergens, which are routinely passed backward into the pharynx to be swallowed into the acidic environment of the stomach. This mucus consists of enzymes, proteins, and inorganic salts. Increased production of mucus occurs with allergic disease, viral infections, bacterial or fungal sinusitis, vasomotor rhinitis, hormonal changes, aging, or exposure to cold.

Postnasal drip may cause a chronically irritated throat, globus sensation, excessive phlegm, or chronic cough. Patients with chronic diffuse sore throat should be asked about postnasal drip and other symptoms of chronic rhinitis or sinusitis including thick or thin rhinorrhea, sneezing, congestion, watery eyes, facial pressure, or a seasonal component to their symptoms. The timing of the sore throat in these cases tends to be worse at night or in the early morning.

Postnasal drip is most frequently associated with allergic rhinitis. Examination findings consistent with allergic rhinitis include enlarged or boggy turbinates, clear secretions that may be either thin or tacky, cobblestoned and hypervascular posterior pharyngeal wall, erythema of the tonsils or tonsillar pillars, pale edema of the posterior larynx, and erythema of the conjunctiva.

Nasal congestion is the sensation of limited air flow through the nose, which waxes and wanes with different exposures and positioning. It differs from nasal obstruction, which is more often a static obstruction attributable to a structural problem such as a deviated nasal septum or nasal mass. Nasal congestion can be seen with rhinitis that is allergic, vasomotor, or infectious in nature. It can also occur after chronic use of intranasal decongestants such as oxymetazoline (Afrin) and phenylephrine (Neosynephrine). The severe nasal congestion that occurs after prolonged use of these over-the-counter nasal sprays is called rhinitis medicamentosa, and will only abate after cessation of the medication.

Both nasal congestion and nasal obstruction can lead to chronic mouth breathing. Mouth breathing bypasses the natural humidification of the nose and is especially problematic at night when dependent nasal congestion occurs. This chronic mouth breathing can lead to a dry and irritated posterior pharynx and complaint of a chronic sore throat.

Saline irrigations and steroid nasal sprays are the first-line therapy for nasal congestion and postnasal drip related to allergic rhinitis. If this is not sufficient, consideration of an antihistamine, either intranasally or orally, may be effective. Ipratropium bromide (Atrovent) is particularly effective for vasomotor rhinitis. Cessation of over-the-counter intranasal decongestants is required for relief of rhinitis medicamentosa. Surgery may be necessary for significant nasal obstruction caused by septal deviation or nasal masses.

Foreign Body

A foreign body in the pharynx may cause a sensation of globus, and the patient may complain of a sore throat if the foreign body causes abrasion or erosion; this is usually a well-localized irritation. Pills are a particularly common irritation for the elderly and those with underlying swallowing or motility disorders. Large pill size and sustained-release pills, especially when taken in the supine position with only a small amount of liquid, are risk factors for pill dysphagia. Fish bones and chicken bones are other common causes of persistent foreign body sensation. Even after the foreign body has passed, inflammation and irritation can persist from the damaged mucosa. This is typically self-limited but sucralfate can provide some additional protection to the mucosa as it heals.

Any persistent foreign body sensation should be evaluated with anteroposterior and lateral neck films. Laryngoscopy may also be required if the suspected foreign body is radiolucent. Pharyngeal and laryngeal foreign bodies require endoscopic removal because of their threat to the patient's airway. Organic material that has passed below the cricopharyngeus can be allowed to continue through the gastrointestinal tract. Batteries must be removed immediately regardless of location, because the acid they contain has the potential to leak and cause a caustic burn in the aerodigestive tract.

Neoplasms

Both benign and malignant neoplasms in the larynx or pharynx can cause globus, irritation, or frank pain in the throat. Benign neoplasms more often cause a sensation of globus without pain or discomfort. Pain is a concerning sign and raises the suspicion of malignancy. Depending on the location, associated symptoms may include dysphagia, odynophagia, otalgia, voice change, weight loss, and lymphadenopathy.

The most common malignant neoplasm in the throat is squamous cell carcinoma and of these, tonsil cancers are the most frequent. Adenocarcinoma, sarcoma, and lymphoma can also occur in the throat and present with sore throat. Patients with persistent sore throats, worsening symptoms, or well-localized pain should be referred to an otolaryngologist for a full evaluation.

REFERENCES

1. Schappert SM, Burt CW. Ambulatory care visits to physician offices, hospital outpatient departments, and emergency departments: United States, 2001-02. Vital Health Stat 13 2006;159:1–66.
2. Ayanruoh S, Waseem M, Quee F, et al. Impact of rapid streptococcal test on antibiotic use in a pediatric emergency department. Pediatr Emerg Care 2009; 25(11):748–50.
3. Finkelstein Y, Bar-Ziv J, Nachmani A, et al. Peritonsillar abscess as a cause of transient velopharyngeal insufficiency. Cleft Palate Craniofac J 1993;30(4):421–8.
4. Bisno A. Acute pharyngitis. N Engl J Med 2001;344(3):205–11.
5. Hoagland RJ. Infectious mononucleosis. Prim Care 1975;2:295–307.
6. Ebell M. Epstein Barr virus infectious mononucleosis. Am Fam Physician 2004; 70(7):1279–87.
7. Ebell MH, White LL, Casault T. A systematic review of the history and physical examination to diagnose influenza. J Am Board Fam Pract 2004;17:1–5.
8. Moscona A. Neuraminidase inhibitors for influenza. N Engl J Med 2005;353(13): 1363–73.
9. Jefferson T, Jones M, Doshi P, et al. Neuraminidase inhibitors for preventing and treating influenza in healthy adults: systematic review and meta-analysis. BMJ 2009;339:b5106.
10. Cooper NJ, Sutton AJ, Abrams KR, et al. Effectiveness of neuraminidase inhibitors in treatment and prevention of influenza A and B: systematic review and meta-analyses of randomised controlled trials. BMJ 2003;326(7401):1235.
11. Glezen WP. Herd protection against influenza. J Clin Virol 2006;37(4):237–43.
12. Available at: http://www.cdc.gov/h1n1flu/recommendations.htm. Accessed January 30, 2010.
13. Komaroff AL, Pas TM, Aronson MD, et al. The prediction of streptococcal pharyngitis in adults. J Gen Intern Med 1986;1:1–7.
14. Walsh BT, Bookheim WW, Johnson RC, et al. Recognition of streptococcal pharyngitis in adults. Arch Intern Med 1975;135(11):1493–7.
15. Marín Cañada J, Cubillo Serna A, Gómez-Escalonilla Cruz N, et al. Is streptococcal pharyngitis diagnosis possible? Aten Primaria 2007;39(7):361–5 [in Spanish].
16. Webb KH. Does culture confirmation of high-sensitivity rapid streptococcal tests make sense? A medical decision analysis. Pediatrics 1998;101(2):E2.
17. Webb KH, Needham CA, Kurtz SR. Use of a high-sensitivity rapid strep test without culture confirmation of negative results: 2 years' experience. J Fam Pract 2000;49(1):34–8.
18. Kaplan EL, Johnson DR, Del Rosario MC, et al. Susceptibility of group A beta-hemolytic streptococci to thirteen antibiotics: examination of 301 strains isolated

in the United States between 1994 and 1997. Pediatr Infect Dis J 1999;18: 1069–72.

19. Shulman ST, Gerber MA. So what's wrong with penicillin for strep throat? Pediatrics 2004;113(6):1816–9.

20. Gerber MA, Baltimore RS, Eaton CB, et al. Prevention of rheumatic fever and diagnosis and treatment of acute Streptococcal pharyngitis: a scientific statement from the American Heart Association Rheumatic Fever, Endocarditis, and Kawasaki Disease Committee of the Council on Cardiovascular Disease in the Young, the Interdisciplinary Council on Functional Genomics and Translational Biology, and the Interdisciplinary Council on Quality of Care and Outcomes Research: endorsed by the American Academy of Pediatrics. Circulation 2009; 119(11):1541–51.

21. Elahi S, Pang G, Ashman R, et al. Enhanced clearance of Candida albicans from the oral cavities of mice following oral administration of Lactobacillus acidophilus. Clin Exp Immunol 2005;141(1):29–36.

22. Hatakka K, Ahola AJ, Yli-Knuuttila H, et al. Probiotics reduce the prevalence of oral candida in the elderly—a randomized controlled trial. J Dent Res 2007; 86(2):125–30.

23. Johnson RF, Stewart MG. The contemporary approach to diagnosis and management of peritonsillar abscess. J Oral Maxillofac Surg 2004;62(12):1545–50.

24. Cherukuri S, Benninger MS. Use of bacteriologic studies in the outpatient management of peritonsillar abscess. Laryngoscope 2002;112(1):18–20.

25. Brook I. Microbiology and management of peritonsillar, retropharyngeal, and parapharyngeal abscesses. Curr Opin Otolaryngol Head Neck Surg 2005;13(3):157–60.

26. Lyon M, Blaivas M. Intraoral ultrasound in the diagnosis and treatment of suspected peritonsillar abscess in the emergency department. Acad Emerg Med 2005;12(1):85–8.

27. Licameli GR, Grillone GA. Inferior pole peritonsillar abscess. Otolaryngol Head Neck Surg 1998;118:95–9.

28. Windfuhr JP, Chen YS. Immediate abscess tonsillectomy—a safe procedure? Auris Nasus Larynx 2001;28(4):323–7.

29. Suzuki M, Ueyama T, Mogi G. Immediate tonsillectomy for peritonsillar abscess. Auris Nasus Larynx 1999;26(3):299–304.

30. Nagy M, Backstrom J. Comparison of the sensitivity of lateral neck radiographs and computed tomography scanning in pediatric deep-neck infections. Laryngoscope 1999;109(5):775–9.

31. Shefelbine SE, Mancuso AA, Gajewski BJ, et al. Pediatric retropharyngeal lymphadenitis: differentiation from retropharyngeal abscess and treatment implications. Otolaryngol Head Neck Surg 2007;136(2):182–8.

32. Malloy KM, Christenson T, Meyer JS, et al. Lack of association of CT findings and surgical drainage in pediatric neck abscesses. Int J Pediatr Otorhinolaryngol 2008;72(2):235–9.

33. Kirse DJ, Roberson DW. Surgical management of retropharyngeal space infections in children. Laryngoscope 2001;111(8):1413–22.

34. Brook I. Microbiology and management of peritonsillar, retropharyngeal, and parapharyngeal abscesses. J Oral Maxillofac Surg 2004;62(12):1545–50.

35. Brook I. Microbiology of retropharyngeal abscesses in children. Am J Dis Child 1987;141(2):202–4.

36. McClay JE, Murray AD, Booth T. Intravenous antibiotic therapy for deep neck abscesses defined by computed tomography. Arch Otolaryngol Head Neck Surg 2003;129(11):1207–12.

37. Page NC, Bauer EM, Lieu JE. Clinical features and treatment of retropharyngeal abscess in children. Otolaryngol Head Neck Surg 2008;138(3):300–6.
38. Frantz TD, Rasgon BM. Acute epiglottitis: changing epidemiologic patterns. Otolaryngol Head Neck Surg 1993;109(3 Pt 1):457–60.
39. Shah RK, Roberson DW, Jones DT. Epiglottitis in the *Haemophilus influenzae* type B vaccine era: changing trends. Laryngoscope 2004;114(3):557–60.
40. Berger G, Landau T, Berger S. The rising incidence of adult acute epiglottitis and epiglottic abscess. Am J Otolaryngol 2003;24(6):374–83.
41. Yazici ZM, Sayin I, Kayhan FT, et al. Laryngopharyngeal reflux might play a role on chronic nonspecific pharyngitis. Eur Arch Otorhinolaryngol 2010;267(4): 571–4.
42. Koufman JA. The Otolaryngologic manifestations of gastroesophageal reflux disease (GERD): a clinical investigation of 225 patients using ambulatory 24-hour pH monitoring and an experimental investigation of the role of acid and pepsin in the development of laryngeal injury. Laryngoscope 1991;101(Suppl 53):1–78.
43. Johnston N, Wells CW, Samuels TL, et al. Pepsin in nonacidic refluxate can damage hypopharyngeal epithelial cells. Ann Otol Rhinol Laryngol 2009;118(9): 677–85.
44. Ofman JJ, Dorn GH, Fennerty MB, et al. The clinical and economic impact of competing management strategies for gastro-oesophageal reflux disease. Aliment Pharmacol Ther 2002;16(2):261–73.

Diagnostic Evaluation and Management of Hoarseness

Ted Mau, MD, PhD

KEYWORDS

• Voice • Dysphonia • Laryngoscopy • Voice evaluation

OVERVIEW

Hoarseness is a common symptom encountered by primary care providers. Hoarseness has a lifetime prevalence of 30%.[1] At any point in time, 3% to 9% of the general population is affected by some type of voice abnormality.[1,2] About 25% or more of the working population in the United States depend on voice as a critical aspect of their jobs.[3] The prevalence of voice problems is higher in people in certain professions, such as teachers, telemarketers, attorneys, and clergy.[1,4] The negative effect of voice disturbance on quality of life and economic productivity is significant and has been well documented.[2,5,6]

Hoarseness can result from a wide spectrum of conditions ranging from the common cold to a malignancy. Because of its prevalence and the multitude of disease processes that can account for it, hoarseness can present a challenge in its diagnosis and management for the general practitioner. This article aims to provide a framework for diagnostic evaluation and assist the provider in determining when a referral to an otolaryngologist may be appropriate. Treatments commonly prescribed for hoarseness are critically examined. This article helps to gain an insight into the assessment of the patient with hoarseness.

WHAT IS HOARSENESS?

Hoarseness is a symptom, not a diagnosis. Hoarseness is a layman's term that is used to describe any deviation from a normal voice quality as perceived by self or others. Although the term hoarseness is suitable as a chief complaint, it is vague and nonspecific. In the same way that dizziness is used to refer to vertigo, light-headedness,

Funding support: None.
Clinical Center for Voice Care, Department of Otolaryngology–Head and Neck Surgery, University of Texas Southwestern Medical Center, 5323 Harry Hines Boulevard, Dallas, TX 75390, USA
E-mail address: ted.mau@utsouthwestern.edu

Med Clin N Am 94 (2010) 945–960
doi:10.1016/j.mcna.2010.05.010
0025-7125/10/$ – see front matter © 2010 Elsevier Inc. All rights reserved.

or postural instability, hoarseness is used by patients to describe a breathy quality to the voice, a roughness, a pitch change, or sometimes some degree of dysarthria. Hoarseness refers to a disturbance in voice. The distinction between voice and speech is important because dysphonia and dysarthria have different underlying causes. Voice refers to the sound produced by the vibrating vocal folds. A voice problem traces its roots to the phonatory mechanism at the vocal fold level. Speech refers to the train of sounds shaped by the pharynx, tongue, oral cavity, and lips to form words and phrases. Most speech disturbances tend to have a central neurologic basis, such as stroke, whereas most voice disturbances tend to arise from problems at the end organ, for example, the vocal folds, or in the peripheral control of the end organ (spasmodic dysphonia [SD] being a notable exception).

To gain an appreciation of the different pathophysiologic mechanisms that could lead to voice disturbance, it is useful to begin with a simple description of voice and how it is produced.

PHYSIOLOGY OF VOICE PRODUCTION

The human voice is produced by passive vibrations of the vocal folds in an air stream, usually on exhalation. The vibrations produce pressure waves that are received by the auditory system and perceived as sound, much like any sound source producing pressure waves that are perceived as the sound of a siren, a French horn, or a cello. Normal human voice production requires several elements:

1. An adequate air stream to initiate and sustain vocal fold vibrations
2. Vocal fold edges that are free from aberrations
3. Vocal folds with normal tissue properties to allow vibrations
4. Optimal posturing of the 2 vocal folds in contact or near contact
5. Proper internal tension of the vocal folds to produce the desired pitch and voice quality.

If normal voice is a series of pressure waves with a certain shape produced by normal vocal folds, then an aberration on the vibrating edge of a vocal fold, a change in the distance between the 2 vibrating edges, or a change in the internal tension of the vocal folds can all change the shape of the pressure waves, which are then perceived as an altered sound or hoarseness. Each of these elements is addressed in turn.

PATHOPHYSIOLOGY OF HOARSENESS

Most cases of hoarseness result from disturbance in one of the elements required for normal voice production as outlined earlier. Major categories of pathologic conditions affecting the voice are explained in terms of the type of problem they cause.

Poor Breath Support

Voice disturbance can occur in the absence of pathologic conditions in the larynx. Inadequate breath support for phonation is common even in healthy individuals. The sound intensity from the glottis can be increased by increasing subglottic pressure either by using better breath support or by posturing the vocal folds together tighter. The former is a natural mechanism, whereas the latter can be pathologic because it increases the mechanical stress on the vocal folds and requires hyperfunction of extralaryngeal musculature that is normally used for swallowing and not phonation. The increased stress on the vocal folds produces a pressed quality to the voice. This condition falls under the broad category of muscle tension dysphonia (MTD).[7–9]

Discrete Vocal Fold Edge Aberrations

This category of diseases is perhaps the most intuitive to appreciate. Discrete vocal fold aberrations can change the pressure waveform of normal voice by preventing full contact of the entire length of the membranous vocal folds, by damping the vocal fold vibration, or both. The most common categories of discrete vocal fold aberrations are discussed.

Benign lesions related to phonotrauma

Vocal fold nodules, polyps, and, to a lesser extent, cysts are formed as the tissue's response to chronically elevated mechanical stress during vocal fold vibrations. Nodules are by definition bilateral and form at the midpoint of the membranous vocal folds, which is the location of the greatest impact. Polyps can be unilateral or bilateral and broad based or pedunculated, with submillimeter size to spanning the entire length of the membranous vocal fold, and can have appearances that vary from translucent to hemorrhagic. Cysts can contain fluid (mucus retention cyst) or can be cellular (epithelial inclusion cyst). The precise differentiation between these types of benign lesions is less important to the generalist than the appreciation that many of these lesions do not require surgical removal. Many lesions resolve or regress sufficiently to improve voice with adequate voice therapy described later.

Papillomas

The vocal folds are the primary site of occurrence for recurrent respiratory papillomatosis. These warts are caused by the human papillomavirus, mostly types 6 and 11. The incidence in US adults is estimated to be 1.8 per 100,000.[10] Although the vast majority of patients have benign disease, malignant transformation is reported to occur in 1.6% of the patients.[11] The primary morbidity for many patients is the need for repeated surgical procedures to control the disease because of its propensity to recur. New office-based methods have been developed in recent years to reduce the cost and time associated with treatments.[12] Some presentations of vocal fold papillomas may be difficult to distinguish from vocal fold polyps without high-quality laryngoscopy. Operative laryngoscopy with magnification is then mandated, with biopsy if the visual appearance is consistent with the papilloma.

Squamous cell carcinoma

A laryngeal malignancy that manifests as hoarseness is a must-not-miss diagnosis. It is not possible to distinguish malignant lesions from benign lesions based on history and auditory perception alone, although a history of smoking should greatly increase the clinician's suspicion for a malignant process. Of all the possible causes of hoarseness, it is this entity that makes laryngoscopy indispensable in the assessment of hoarseness that does not resolve in a short amount of time.

The most common laryngeal malignancy is squamous cell carcinoma (SCC). The annual incidences of SCC in the United States are 6.2 and 1.3 in 100,000 men and women, respectively,[13] with approximately 56% originating on the vocal folds[14] and therefore would manifest first as hoarseness. Because the survival and treatment morbidity of laryngeal SCC correlate with the extent of the disease, timely diagnosis and treatment is of paramount importance.

Leukoplakia

A range of vocal fold lesions appear as white plaques and represent a spectrum of hyperplasia, metaplasia, and dysplasia. These lesions are generally considered to be potentially premalignant, but their appearance does not correlate with malignant potential. More than half of the lesions biopsied in a large series showed no dysplasia.[15] The annual incidences in the United States are 10.2 and 2.1 per 100,000 men and women, respectively.[16] A variety of causative factors have been proposed to contribute to the development of leukoplakia, including tobacco and alcohol use, occupational exposure to irritants, and laryngopharyngeal reflux (LPR).[17] Once identified by laryngoscopy, leukoplakia in the absence of other signs suggestive of invasive carcinoma can be observed over a month of conservative measures consisting of cessation of tobacco and alcohol use, optimization of vocal hygiene, and acid suppression therapy.[17] If the lesion does not regress and/or if hoarseness worsens, a biopsy should be undertaken.

Diffuse Change in Vocal Fold Tissue Vibratory Properties

The human vocal folds have a unique layered structure unparalleled to any other species. The ability to communicate with a range of inflections and with songs relies on the viscoelastic properties of each of the layers. To produce an intended voice, the vocal folds need to posture at a specific length with a defined amount of internal tension. In addition, the most superficial layer of the vocal fold lamina propria (SLLP) must remain supple to allow self-sustained oscillation in the order of 100 to 400 Hz. Many disease processes can affect the suppleness or the viscoelastic properties of the SLLP.

Most conditions that result in diffuse change in vocal fold tissue do so by causing vocal fold inflammation. Inflammation increases the water and cellular contents of the SLLP, resulting in lowered pitch, roughness of voice, and increased energy necessary to initiate and sustain phonation.

Upper respiratory tract infection

Acute laryngitis, as part of a viral upper respiratory tract infection (URTI), is probably the most common cause of hoarseness. Acute laryngitis tends to be self-limited and should resolve with other symptoms of the URTI. Although over-the-counter remedies for URTIs abound, the best management for URTI-associated laryngitis consists of aggressive hydration, abstinence from caffeine and alcohol for their diuretic effects, relative voice rest, and avoidance of decongestants. Decongestants are indicated if nasal obstruction is a significant symptom but should be avoided otherwise because of their systemic drying effect.

If the voice change occurs without any other symptoms of a URTI, a diagnosis other than acute laryngitis should be considered.

Reflux

Reflux of gastric contents into the larynx, variably called LPR or extraesophageal reflux, is one of the most commonly ascribed and the most controversial causes for hoarseness. LPR causes vocal fold inflammation and therefore voice change.[18] The controversy is over making the diagnosis of LPR based on signs and symptoms. Because LPR is thought to be highly prevalent, affecting as much as 30% of the population,[19] it is not straightforward to establish a causal relationship between voice change, which is also prevalent and has many possible causes, and LPR, simply because they can coexist without a direct relationship. Although LPR should be assessed and considered in every patient with throat complaints, including hoarseness, it may have become overdiagnosed because of voice change.[20,21]

Allergies

Allergic rhinitis has long been recognized to affect the voice. Increased nasal drainage, altered mucus production, and general upper airway irritation can have a secondary effect on the vocal folds.[22] In addition, allergens may exert a direct effect on the laryngeal mucosa.[23] Frequently, the voice change associated with allergic rhinitis is caused by its treatments. Systemic antihistamines, especially the first-generation type, have a drying effect. Systemic decongestants, another common component of over-the-counter allergy relief drugs, also tend to dehydrate the vocal fold mucosa. To minimize these undesired side effects, topical nasal steroids are recommended as first-line therapy.

Smoking
Chronic smoke exposure causes edema of the SLLP, also called Reinke edema or polypoid corditis. The increased mass of the SLLP leads to a lowered pitch and a rough quality to the voice, especially noticeable in female smokers. Cessation of smoking does not necessarily lead to complete resolution of the edema. Voice change in patients with preexisting Reinke edema can signal an acute increase in the size of a swollen vocal fold (eg, from severe coughing). However, any voice change in a smoker necessitates laryngoscopy to rule out a neoplastic process.

Hypothyroidism
Voice disturbance is thought to be one of the symptoms of hypothyroidism. The mechanism is presumed to involve vocal fold edema, although the precise mechanism is unknown. If laryngoscopy reveals mild, diffuse edema of the vocal folds in a nonsmoker, it is reasonable to check thyroid-stimulating hormone level to rule out hypothyroidism.

Inappropriate Posturing of the Vocal Folds
Most problems in this category involve underadduction of the vocal folds, although overadduction can also cause voice disturbance. Normal voice production requires mechanically stable juxtaposition of the 2 vocal folds in near contact. The vocal folds are brought into apposition by the intrinsic laryngeal muscles, which act on the cricoarytenoid joint and the cricothyroid joint to position the 2 vocal folds in a desired phonatory position. Underadduction, as in unilateral vocal fold paralysis, in general produces a "breathy" voice. Overadduction, as in MTD, results in a pressed voice.

Vocal fold paralysis
The most common cause of unilateral vocal fold paralysis is iatrogenic, from surgeries in the vicinity of the recurrent laryngeal nerve (RLN).[24] The next most common category is idiopathic. The third most common cause is malignancy, with lung cancer accounting for a majority.[24] Intubation accounts for 4% to 7% of malignancies, although this could be from either neuropraxia of the RLN or cricoarytenoid joint dysfunction. A weak, breathy voice should therefore prompt the examiner to review these common causes. Diagnosis of vocal fold paralysis requires laryngoscopic finding of a vocal fold without active mobility but with a small degree of passive mobility to exclude joint fixation. In some cases, laryngeal electromyography may be indicated to distinguish between the 2 possibilities.

Functional dysphonia
Functional dysphonia comprises a broad category of voice disorders without an organic origin. The vocal folds are normal in appearance and have normal mobility with nonphonatory tasks. However, the fine balance of the intrinsic laryngeal muscle system is disturbed so that hyperfunction results, producing a pressed voice, a breathy voice, or no voice at all.

Two common subsets of functional dysphonia are worthy of mention. MTD is characterized by hyperfunction of the intrinsic laryngeal muscles.[9] Hyperfunctional posturing of the supraglottic structures is a common laryngoscopic finding.[7,25] Tenderness on palpation of the thyrohyoid muscles as a sign of chronic hyperfunction and fatigue is also seen on external neck examination. A pressed voice results from overadduction of the vocal folds. Psychogenic functional dysphonia or aphonia can also involve hyperfunction of the laryngeal muscles and is so termed to reflect a predominant psychological cause. These 2 subsets of functional voice disorders are not necessarily mutually exclusive. Both voice disorders are treated by therapy with a speech-language pathologist with expertise in voice disorders, although some patients with psychogenic dysphonia may benefit from concurrent psychological treatment.

SD

Frequently incorrectly called spastic dysphonia, SD is a neurologic disorder specific to the speaking voice. The normally controlled posturing of the vocal folds in speech is disrupted by adductory or abductory spasms that produce the characteristic voice breaks heard in adductor SD (Audio 1) or abductor SD (Audio 2). Unlike most of the other conditions that cause hoarseness, which rely on laryngoscopy for definitive diagnosis, the diagnosis of SD is largely made based on auditory perceptual characteristics by experienced listeners. Although without a cure, SD has been treated successfully with periodic injections of botulinum toxin into the affected laryngeal muscles, as well as by other surgical techniques.

Essential tremor

Essential tremor occurs or worsens with sustained posture. Patients with essential tremor of the voice may or may not have tremors affecting other parts of the body. As with SD, a diagnosis of vocal tremor is largely made by auditory perception but can be confirmed by laryngoscopy to visualize the structures involved in the rhythmic movements. Isolated vocal tremors are sometimes misdiagnosed as SD, because the tremors can lead to phonatory interruptions that are perceived as voice breaks.

ASSESSMENT

A useful diagnostic approach to hoarseness is to gather specific pieces of information, each of which contributes to a final impression of a pretest probability of whether the condition responsible for hoarseness fits into 1 of the 3 categories:

- Temporary or reversible in nature and resolves spontaneously or with appropriate medical therapy (eg, URTI, reflux, allergies)
- Chronic and benign, requiring nonurgent otolaryngology referral and definitive diagnosis (eg, vocal fold nodules and polyps, functional dysphonia, SD, vocal tremor)
- Potentially serious, requiring timely referral and possible further workup (eg, vocal fold paralysis, primary laryngeal malignancy).

Much of the information needed to form such a clinical impression is gleamed from the history.

History

Onset, duration, and progression

As with most medical conditions, a voice problem that began many years ago and has remained stable for sometime is less likely to require urgent intervention than the one that began a few weeks ago and has continued to worsen. However, this simple rule of thumb needs to be applied with caution because the cause of hoarseness can be highly varied. A voice change that developed suddenly 4 weeks ago and has left a patient almost aphonic (eg, functional dysphonia) may be less serious than a voice change that began a year ago and has only slowly progressed (eg, a vocal fold SCC). It is always useful to query the circumstances of onset, specifically whether the voice change occurred in the context of the following:

- *A URTI.* Voice disturbance is common in URTIs because the vocal folds become inflamed as part of the overall disease process. However, the voice should normalize within 1 to 2 weeks of the resolution of other symptoms. If the voice remains abnormal for more than 3 to 4 weeks after resolution of other symptoms, including cough, either chronic changes have developed on the vocal folds or the voice production mechanism has remained dysfunctional.
- *Trauma to the larynx or RLNs.* Did the voice change after surgery in the neck or chest? Was the patient intubated for any reason? What was the timing of the voice change relative to the time of surgery or intubation?
- *Period of increased vocal demand or episode of voice abuse/overuse.* Phono-trauma in either case can lead to vocal fold hemorrhage and polyp or nodule formation. Typical scenarios for increased vocal demand include an increase in teaching load, a change to a job involving more presentations and meetings, or a new role outside of a singer's typical vocal range. Typical scenarios of episodes of voice abuse or overuse include yelling at sporting events or new coughing fits.
- *Time of emotional distress.* The onset of functional voice disorders, psychogenic or not, often coincides with a time of emotional distress. Certain neurologic conditions affecting the voice, such as SD or vocal tremor, are exacerbated by stress, and patients who experience the symptoms for the first time may well develop the first manifestation of the condition during a time of stress.

Change in voice quality
The nature of the change in voice quality provides further clues to the possible causes, although most patients may not be able to differentiate one voice quality from another. Often, patients report the development of a raspy voice. If a roughness of the voice is meant, that is, the loss of smoothness and clarity, some type of vocal fold edge aber-ration may have formed. The development of a breathy or weak voice suggests hypo-adduction of the vocal folds and should lead to suspicion of vocal fold paralysis. A tightness of the voice may reflect MTD, SD, or even vocal tremor. Patients who have more vocal awareness may report a change in pitch.

Variation with daily activity or voice use
Does the patient wake up with a normal voice that worsens as the day progresses? Does the voice quality worsen with use, or is it poor even without much use of voice? Does the voice recover with rest? If the voice quality starts normal but worsens with use, the underlying problem is probably not a fixed anatomic abnormality such as a vocal fold lesion. On the other hand, subtle weakness of the vocal folds (vocal fold paresis) may not manifest as a change in voice quality but as new vocal fatigue with use.

Presence of normal voice
Does the patient have periods of normal voice in between the periods of poor voice? When was the last time the patient had a normal voice? If a normal voice is present for some time, it argues against a fixed anatomic or neurologic abnormality and offers some degree of reassurance to the clinician. A patient who has had voice disturbance

for 6 months and has not had a normal voice for 3 months requires more urgent assessment than a patient whose dysphonia began around the same time but who had 5 hours of normal voice 2 days ago.

Association with other symptoms

Does the patient have associated symptoms? Does the voice tend to worsen when the patient's allergy or reflux symptoms flare up? Does the voice improve when the patient's allergy or reflux is treated? Did the hoarseness develop after a new chronic cough started? If so, the assessment may need to include targeted questioning for possible causes of cough. The converse history is also useful. If the patient's hoarseness occurs in the absence of itchy and watery eyes, sneezing, cough, and clear rhinorrhea, it is probably not related to allergies. If the hoarseness occurs in a patient without any classic symptoms of gastroesophageal reflux disease (GERD) (heartburn, regurgitation, acid taste in back of mouth) and without other symptoms commonly attributed to LPR (globus sensation, throat clearing, cough), then the hoarseness is probably not due to reflux.

Past medical and surgical history

Has the patient had recent surgery in the neck or chest? Has the patient had neck or chest surgery in the past, and if so, was there voice change afterward? Some cases of vocal fold paralysis remain undiagnosed because of favorable compensation from the contralateral vocal fold. Is there any history of intubation?

Does the patient have known or subclinical hypothyroidism? Although uncommon, several rheumatic diseases can involve the larynx, including rheumatoid arthritis, Wegener granulomatosis, sarcoidosis, amyloidosis, and systemic lupus erythematosus.

Tobacco use

Smoking is the number one risk factor for the development of laryngeal cancer. A past or current history of smoking in a patient with voice change should alert the clinician and lower the threshold for laryngoscopy. The risk of malignancy declines with cessation of smoking but does not return near the level of that of nonsmokers until 15 years after cessation.[26]

Occupation

The occupation and extent of work-related voice use should be established for every patient with hoarseness. These data inform the clinician about the effect of the voice problem on the patient's quality of life and the ability to carry out his or her job. Patients with a severe voice problem may be at risk of losing employment if a normal voice is crucial to their job description. Across countries, teachers consistently emerge as most likely to seek medical attention for a voice problem.[27] Other high-risk occupations include working as counselors, attorneys, clergy, and singers. If the clinician determines that the voice problem significantly affects the patient's ability to work, expeditious referral for laryngoscopy and voice assessment is advised. Singers who present with a new or persistent voice problem benefit from evaluation by otolaryngologists with expertise in care of the professional voice. Although these particular occupations are risk factors for voice problems, patients with jobs not typically considered high risk for developing voice problems are not immune from voice misuse in work or nonwork environments.

These elements of history help the clinician to form an overall impression of the potential seriousness of the underlying condition responsible for the voice disturbance. However, these are general guidelines. The impression must be confirmed or modified by further assessment.

Clinical Examination

Auditory perceptual evaluation

A trained listener can narrow the differential diagnosis for an abnormal voice based on the acoustic qualities of the voice. A breathy voice (Audio 3) suggests glottic insufficiency from hypoadduction of the vocal folds or a decrease in the tone of the thyroarytenoid muscle. A pressed or constricted voice (Audio 4) implies hyperadduction or hyperfunction. A rough voice (Audio 5) suggests vocal fold edge aberrations or a diffuse change in the vibratory properties as in inflammation. A weak or asthenic voice suggests vocal fold weakness or decreased pulmonary drive. A persistently elevated pitch is often consistent with a functional disorder (Audio 4). Diplophonia (Audio 3), which refers to simultaneous sound at 2 different pitches, results from vibrations of the 2 vocal folds at separate frequencies and can result from unilateral vocal fold paralysis, a mass lesion on one vocal fold, or any type of asymmetry between the vocal folds.

Physical examination

In addition to a complete head and neck examination, particular attention should be given to possible thyromegaly, cervical lymphadenopathy, obvious asymmetry in the neck, and surgical scars. Moisture of the oral cavity's mucous membrane is a useful surrogate indicator of the adequacy of vocal fold hydration. The oropharynx should be inspected for posterior pharyngeal wall erythema or cobblestoning. Although these signs are nonspecific, they are reflective of mucosal irritation and may be consistent with URTI, possible nasal drainage, or possible high reflux.

Laryngoscopy

It should be obvious from the earlier enumeration of possible causes for hoarseness that most conditions cannot be definitively diagnosed without visualizing the vocal folds and the rest of the larynx. The value of laryngoscopy in the diagnosis of hoarseness has been addressed in a clinical practice guideline on hoarseness.[28] Practically, the most important reason to visualize the larynx in hoarseness is to rule out a malignancy. Timely laryngoscopy helps to establish the diagnosis and avoid treatment delay. In addition to identifying benign or malignant mass lesions, inspection of the larynx should document the mobility of the vocal folds and arytenoids, presence of thick mucus, and presence or absence of signs consistent with mucosal irritation, such as LPR. Laryngoscopy is helpful even in conditions in which the diagnosis is made largely from auditory perception, such as SD and vocal tremor. In these cases, laryngoscopy serves to rule out coexisting anatomic abnormalities such as vocal fold lesions. Findings from laryngoscopy can also direct treatment by identifying asymmetry in vocal fold spasms or the direction and the anatomic substrates of the tremor.

The larynx can be visualized by several methods. The simplest method in terms of equipment need is indirect mirror laryngoscopy, which has been practiced for more than a century. A view of the larynx is obtained with a headlight illuminating the larynx via a round mirror positioned anterior to the uvula. This method is still used by a small number of general practitioners. The view obtained is clear but brief and mostly serves to rule out obvious lesions. Some patients' anatomy does not allow complete visualization of the vocal folds.

If indirect laryngoscopy proves inadequate, laryngoscopy can be performed with a transnasal flexible scope. This is the most widely used method today and is not only ubiquitous in otolaryngology offices but also used by some clinicians in other specialties.

Laryngeal videostroboscopy

Laryngoscopy performed with a constant-source light cannot assess the vibratory properties of the vocal folds or visualize small lesions that interfere with vibrations. If a patient has hoarseness and laryngoscopy does not show obvious anatomic abnormalities, videostroboscopy is indicated to assess the vocal fold vibratory properties. It should be performed by a clinician skilled in the performance and interpretation of the video examination. Conditions that should be further assessed by videostroboscopy include but are not limited to vocal fold polyps and cysts, vocal fold hemorrhage, and subtle vocal fold weakness or hypoadduction.

MANAGEMENT

Treatment of hoarseness does not and cannot follow a predetermined algorithm because the treatment must be tailored for the particular diagnosis. For example, treatment of acute laryngitis in a vocal performer may include administration of oral or intramuscular steroids, which would be inappropriate for a patient with SD or MTD. The following section examines some treatments commonly prescribed for the symptom of hoarseness and underlines the appropriate and inappropriate approaches.

Antireflux Medication

Antireflux medication, in particular proton pump inhibitors (PPIs), is widely prescribed by internists and otolaryngologists for the treatment of the symptom of hoarseness. This practice has become widespread since the connection between LPR and throat complaints was highlighted almost 2 decades ago.[18] Few investigators would debate that the reflux of acidic content into the larynx can cause sufficient inflammation of the vocal folds to cause voice disturbance. What remains controversial is how often voice disturbance is actually caused by acid reflux.[20]

The clinical practice guideline on hoarseness, which provides evidence-based recommendations, recommends against the routine prescription of antireflux medication for the treatment of the symptom of hoarseness without signs or symptoms of GERD or laryngeal findings consistent with laryngitis.[28] This guideline in itself is somewhat controversial, because LPR is regarded by many investigators as an entity that is distinct from GERD, so signs or symptoms of GERD should have no bearing on the LPR symptom of hoarseness. Also, there is no universal agreement on what constitutes signs of laryngitis, which tend to be nonspecific. The guideline also cites the risks associated with prolonged (eg, >3 months) use of PPIs and histamine2 receptor antagonists (H2RAs) as a factor in its recommendation.

There are several other arguments against the routine use of antireflux medication for hoarseness:

1. *Voice complaints in the absence of other symptoms of LPR may not be due to LPR.* In the author's experience at a tertiary referral voice center, patients who present with voice disturbance and no other symptoms of LPR (eg, chronic cough, throat clearing, globus sensation) or of GERD (eg, heartburn, regurgitation) do not tend to respond to PPI therapy. Most of these patients have either a constricted voice or poor breath support or both on auditory perceptual evaluation and evidence of chronic muscle tension of the extralaryngeal musculature on physical examination. Many of these patients have MTD and often respond favorably to voice therapy. The caveat is that this experience is anecdotal, shared by some but not all clinicians at other tertiary referral centers. The nonuniformity of anecdotal experience reflects the inherent individual biases in the greater reflux debate.

2. *Acid reflux can be a coexisting but not a causative condition.* Acid reflux is common. In a local population study in the United States, approximately 40% of the patients experienced heartburn on a monthly basis.[29] LPR is estimated to affect as many as 30% of Americans.[19] When this potential cause for voice disturbance has such high prevalence in the general population, it is expected to be present in a large number of patients with a particular symptom such as hoarseness simply based on chance alone.[30] Causation is difficult to prove. Clinicians rely on symptom questionnaires such as the reflux symptom index[31] and laryngoscopic signs[32] to determine whether there is a high probability of presence of reflux, but laryngoscopy findings have been found to be nonspecific,[33–35] which is another area of great controversy.

3. *Nonacid reflux may be responsible.* There is a growing body of literature supporting the role of nonacid reflux in causing symptoms that are commonly attributed to acidic LPR.[36] The agents postulated to mediate tissue damage in nonacid reflux include pepsin and bile. Much of the evidence supporting pepsin damage so far has been derived from in vitro work,[37,38] and a link to clinical relevance has not been firmly established. However, the idea of nonacid components of the refluxate causing laryngeal inflammation and therefore throat symptoms seems increasingly valid. This theory would partly explain the high nonresponse rate (approaching 50%) of acid suppression therapy for LPR symptoms in some studies.[39] It is highly likely that nonacid reflux is responsible for vocal fold inflammation and therefore hoarseness in a subset of patients. Because PPIs and H_2RAs do not reduce nonacid reflux, they are not expected to be of benefit in these individuals.

Despite concerns with the possible overuse of antireflux medication for hoarseness,[20] PPIs do have an important role when used appropriately. The clinical practice guideline states that antireflux treatment is an option for patients with hoarseness and signs of chronic laryngitis. Because the signs of chronic laryngitis are somewhat observer dependent and nonspecific, the clinician must incorporate other measures to arrive at some estimation of the pretest probability that acid reflux is at least partially responsible for the symptom of hoarseness. These measures may rely on the presence or absence of other symptoms commonly associated with GERD and/or LPR, as previously mentioned. Patients with multiple symptoms in either group may have a high probability of GERD and/or LPR. For these patients, it is reasonable to begin empiric PPI therapy, provided that the patients are followed up to determine the effect. In these cases, the author uses PPI as a diagnostic tool. Do the symptoms improve or resolve on PPI therapy? More importantly, does the hoarseness improve? It is not uncommon for patients to report significant reduction in heartburn without an improvement in hoarseness.

The adequacy of a trial of acid suppression therapy is defined by its dose, duration, time of administration, and patient compliance. There is no universal agreement on what constitutes an adequate dose and length of therapy, but the PPI dosage has been suggested to be twice daily for at least 4 months.[40] The time of administration is important and is frequently neglected by patients and some prescribing clinicians.[41] PPIs exert their effect by inactivating gastric parietal cell proton pumps. Optimal acid suppression is achieved when PPIs are taken before a meal to allow absorption and accumulation of the drug before the proton pumps are activated.[42] Patients should be instructed to take the medication 30 to 60 minutes before a designated meal.

Corticosteroids

The premise of treating the symptom of hoarseness with corticosteroids lies in their antiinflammatory property and the assumption that hoarseness implies laryngeal inflammation. This practice has no evidence-based support. The clinical practice guideline recommends against the routine use of oral steroids to treat hoarseness based on the preponderance of harm over benefit.[28] The increased incidence of adverse events associated with orally administered steroids is well documented, whereas evidence to show benefit for routine use is lacking.

Steroids do have an important role in the armamentarium of a specialist taking care of a voice professional. The most typical scenario in which steroids are used is in the case of acute laryngitis, shortly before a public event in which voice use cannot be avoided. In this case, steroids are the only means to quickly reduce vocal fold inflammation to allow vocal performance. Inflammation of the vocal folds should be verified by laryngoscopy. The steroids can be given orally if the performing event is more than 2 days away. If the event is to take place sooner, a combination of short- and long-acting intramuscular corticosteroids can be administered in a single dose. Potential risks and adverse events must be explained to the patient and preferably documented in an informed consent.

Antibiotics

Antibiotics compose another category of medications that are frequently inappropriately prescribed for hoarseness. The clinical practice guideline contains a strong recommendation against their use.[28] The most common cause of hoarseness seen in the medical setting is URTI, and most URTIs are viral in nature. A Cochrane review showed no benefit of antibiotics in the treatment of acute laryngitis.[43]

Voice Therapy

Voice therapy consists of various vocalization and breathing exercises designed to retrain the laryngeal muscles to produce the best sound in the least traumatic way. It also incorporates education to improve vocal hygiene and avoid harmful vocal behaviors.[44] Voice therapy is effective in improving vocal function in a variety of voice disorders.[2] Voice therapy is, for the most part, the only option for voice disturbance without an underlying anatomic or neurologic abnormality, such as MTD. Voice therapy is often the first-line therapy for certain benign vocal fold lesions such as nodules, polyps, or cysts.[45] Even for SD, a focal dystonia typically treated with botulinum toxin injections, concurrent voice therapy has been shown to be of benefit.[46] Lee Silverman voice therapy, a specific type of voice therapy, is the most effective treatment of hypophonia seen in patients with Parkinson disease.[47] Voice therapy is also an important adjunct to any vocal fold surgery to optimize vocal outcome and facilitate healing.[44]

Voice therapy should be prescribed only when a diagnosis or a provisional diagnosis has been made to explain the symptom of hoarseness. Voice therapy cannot be prescribed simply because a patient has persistent hoarseness. Because the diagnosis of the underlying cause almost always involves laryngoscopy, voice therapy should not be prescribed without laryngoscopy to verify the nature of the problem.[28]

Voice therapy is ideally performed by a speech-language pathologist with additional postgraduate training in the treatment of voice disorders. Most voice therapies involve 1 to 2 therapy sessions weekly for 6 to 10 weeks.[44]

HOARSENESS IN THE AGED POPULATION

Voice change in the elderly deserves additional attention. Hoarseness in the aged population is a relatively common but undertreated condition. Surveys show a 20% to 29% prevalence of self-reported voice problems in several senior independent living communities.[48–50] Many of those surveyed believed that difficulty with the voice is a natural part of aging,[50] and only 15% to 20% sought care for their voice problem.[48,49] Voice disturbance in this population, possibly combined with declining auditory function, has a demonstrated–negative effect on social function and quality of life.[51]

It is important to resist the temptation to simply attribute a voice problem in the older population to the aging process. Most voice problems in this population are not caused by physiologic aging per se. In most patients, pathologic conditions such as central neurologic disorders, benign vocal fold lesions, inflammatory disorders, neoplasia, and laryngeal paralysis are found.[52] Only about 1 in 5 patients had age-related vocal fold atrophy to account for the voice change.[53]

REFERRAL

The decision to refer otolaryngologic assessment depends on the clinician's index of suspicion that is largely determined by the history of the patient. Specialty referral is unnecessary if the condition underlying the hoarseness is thought to be most likely temporary or reversible in nature and resolves spontaneously or with appropriate medical therapy. In these cases, it is vital that the patient understands the importance of a timely follow-up visit to verify symptom resolution or to assess response to treatment. Referral is indicated when the underlying condition is unclear or the hoarseness fails to resolve. In general, any voice change that persists for more than 2 to 4 weeks warrants further assessment by laryngoscopy, with the chief purpose of ruling out a malignancy.[54–56] The clinical practice guideline recommends laryngoscopy when hoarseness "fails to resolve by a maximum of three months after onset, or irrespective of duration if a serious underlying cause is suspected." The 3-months time frame was selected as a safety net approach to allow time for the patient to follow-up with the primary care provider and then to be assessed by an otolaryngologist within that period. This time frame is meant to be an upper limit and not the recommended time to wait before making a referral. A small vocal fold cancer that causes hoarseness can almost always be visualized by laryngoscopy at the onset. A delay of 3 months in diagnosis can translate into a significant reduction in the 5-year survival rate.

SUMMARY

Hoarseness is a symptom with a wide variety of possible underlying causes, ranging from the mundane to malignancy. Targeted history can assist the clinician to grossly stratify the problem in terms of need or timing for laryngoscopy and for possible otolaryngologic referral. Laryngoscopy is required for diagnosis of the underlying cause in most cases. Given its negative effect on quality of life and personal productivity, persistent hoarseness should be addressed even when not caused by a serious pathologic process.

APPENDIX: SUPPLEMENTARY MATERIAL

Supplementary material can be found, in the online version, at DOI:10.1016/j.mcna.2010.05.010.

REFERENCES

1. Roy N, Merrill RM, Gray SD, et al. Voice disorders in the general population: prevalence, risk factors, and occupational impact. Laryngoscope 2005;115:1988.
2. Ramig LO, Verdolini K. Treatment efficacy: voice disorders. J Speech Lang Hear Res 1998;41:S101.

3. Titze IR, Lemke J, Montequin D. Populations in the U.S. workforce who rely on voice as a primary tool of trade: a preliminary report. J Voice 1997;11:254.
4. Roy N, Merrill RM, Thibeault S, et al. Prevalence of voice disorders in teachers and the general population. J Speech Lang Hear Res 2004;47:281.
5. Cohen SM, Dupont WD, Courey MS. Quality-of-life impact of non-neoplastic voice disorders: a meta-analysis. Ann Otol Rhinol Laryngol 2006;115:128.
6. Benninger MS, Ahuja AS, Gardner G, et al. Assessing outcomes for dysphonic patients. J Voice 1998;12:540.
7. Morrison MD, Rammage LA. Muscle misuse voice disorders: description and classification. Acta Otolaryngol 1993;113:428.
8. Rosen CA, Murry T. Nomenclature of voice disorders and vocal pathology. Otolaryngol Clin North Am 2000;33:1035.
9. Altman KW, Atkinson C, Lazarus C. Current and emerging concepts in muscle tension dysphonia: a 30-month review. J Voice 2005;19:261.
10. Derkay CS, Wiatrak B. Recurrent respiratory papillomatosis: a review. Laryngoscope 2008;118:1236.
11. Dedo HH, Yu KC. CO(2) laser treatment in 244 patients with respiratory papillomas. Laryngoscope 2001;111:1639.
12. Zeitels SM, Burns JA. Office-based laryngeal laser surgery with local anesthesia. Curr Opin Otolaryngol Head Neck Surg 2007;15:141.
13. National Cancer Institute website. Surveillance epidemiology and end results. Available at: http://www.seer.cancer.gov/statfacts/html/laryn.html. Accessed March 27, 2010.
14. Shah JP, Karnell LH, Hoffman HT, et al. Patterns of care for cancer of the larynx in the United States. Arch Otolaryngol Head Neck Surg 1997;123:475.
15. Isenberg JS, Crozier DL, Dailey SH. Institutional and comprehensive review of laryngeal leukoplakia. Ann Otol Rhinol Laryngol 2008;117:74.
16. Bouquot JE, Gnepp DR. Laryngeal precancer: a review of the literature, commentary, and comparison with oral leukoplakia. Head Neck 1991;13:488.
17. Zeitels SM, Casiano RR, Gardner GM, et al. Management of common voice problems: committee report. Otolaryngol Head Neck Surg 2002;126:333.
18. Koufman JA. The otolaryngologic manifestations of gastroesophageal reflux disease (GERD): a clinical investigation of 225 patients using ambulatory 24-hour pH monitoring and an experimental investigation of the role of acid and pepsin in the development of laryngeal injury. Laryngoscope 1991;101:1.
19. Koufman JA. Laryngopharyngeal reflux 2002: a new paradigm of airway disease. Ear Nose Throat J 2002;81:2.
20. Cohen SM, Garrett CG. Hoarseness: is it really laryngopharyngeal reflux? Laryngoscope 2008;118:363.
21. Garrett CG, Cohen SM. Otolaryngological perspective on patients with throat symptoms and laryngeal irritation. Curr Gastroenterol Rep 2008;10:195.
22. Cohn JR, Spiegel JR, Sataloff RT. Vocal disorders and the professional voice user: the allergist's role. Ann Allergy Asthma Immunol 1995;74:363.
23. Dworkin JP, Reidy PM, Stachler RJ, et al. Effects of sequential Dermatophagoides pteronyssinus antigen stimulation on anatomy and physiology of the larynx. Ear Nose Throat J 2009;88:793.
24. Rosenthal LH, Benninger MS, Deeb RH. Vocal fold immobility: a longitudinal analysis of etiology over 20 years. Laryngoscope 1864;117:2007.
25. Koufman JA, Blalock PD. Functional voice disorders. Otolaryngol Clin North Am 1991;24:1059.

26. Falk RT, Pickle LW, Brown LM, et al. Effect of smoking and alcohol consumption on laryngeal cancer risk in coastal Texas. Cancer Res 1989;49:4024.
27. Verdolini K, Ramig LO. Review: occupational risks for voice problems. Logoped Phoniatr Vocol 2001;26:37.
28. Schwartz SR, Cohen SM, Dailey SH, et al. Clinical practice guideline: hoarseness. Otolaryngol Head Neck Surg 2009;141:S1.
29. Locke GR 3rd, Talley NJ, Fett SL, et al. Prevalence and clinical spectrum of gastro-esophageal reflux: a population-based study in Olmsted County, Minnesota. Gastroenterology 1997;112:1448.
30. Long MD, Shaheen NJ. Epidemiology of extraesophageal reflux disease. In: Vaezi MF, editor. Extraesophageal reflux. San Diego (CA): Plural Publishing; 2009. p. 1–18.
31. Belafsky PC, Postma GN, Koufman JA. Validity and reliability of the reflux symptom index (RSI). J Voice 2002;16:274.
32. Belafsky PC, Postma GN, Koufman JA. The validity and reliability of the reflux finding score (RFS). Laryngoscope 2001;111:1313.
33. Hicks DM, Ours TM, Abelson TI, et al. The prevalence of hypopharynx findings associated with gastroesophageal reflux in normal volunteers. J Voice 2002;16:564.
34. Milstein CF, Charbel S, Hicks DM, et al. Prevalence of laryngeal irritation signs associated with reflux in asymptomatic volunteers: impact of endoscopic technique (rigid vs. flexible laryngoscope). Laryngoscope 2005;115:2256.
35. Branski RC, Bhattacharyya N, Shapiro J. The reliability of the assessment of endoscopic laryngeal findings associated with laryngopharyngeal reflux disease. Laryngoscope 2002;112:1019.
36. Sharma N, Agrawal A, Freeman J, et al. An analysis of persistent symptoms in acid-suppressed patients undergoing impedance-pH monitoring. Clin Gastroenterol Hepatol 2008;6:521.
37. Johnston N, Wells CW, Samuels TL, et al. Pepsin in nonacidic refluxate can damage hypopharyngeal epithelial cells. Ann Otol Rhinol Laryngol 2009;118:677.
38. Samuels TL, Johnston N. Pepsin as a causal agent of inflammation during nonacidic reflux. Otolaryngol Head Neck Surg 2009;141:559.
39. Long MD, Shaheen NJ. Extra-esophageal GERD: clinical dilemma of epidemiology versus clinical practice. Curr Gastroenterol Rep 2007;9:195.
40. Vaezi MF, Hicks DM, Abelson TI, et al. Laryngeal signs and symptoms and gastroesophageal reflux disease (GERD): a critical assessment of cause and effect association. Clin Gastroenterol Hepatol 2003;1:333.
41. Chheda NN, Postma GN. Patient compliance with proton pump inhibitor therapy in an otolaryngology practice. Ann Otol Rhinol Laryngol 2008;117:670.
42. Hatlebakk JG, Katz PO, Camacho-Lobato L, et al. Proton pump inhibitors: better acid suppression when taken before a meal than without a meal. Aliment Pharmacol Ther 2000;14:1267.
43. Reveiz L, Cardona AF, Ospina EG. Antibiotics for acute laryngitis in adults. Cochrane Database Syst Rev 2007;2:CD004783.
44. Verdolini K. Guide to vocology. Iowa City (IA): National Center for Voice and Speech; 1998.
45. Cohen SM, Garrett CG. Utility of voice therapy in the management of vocal fold polyps and cysts. Otolaryngol Head Neck Surg 2007;136:742.
46. Murry T, Woodson GE. Combined-modality treatment of adductor spasmodic dysphonia with botulinum toxin and voice therapy. J Voice 1995;9:460.

47. Fox CM, Ramig LO, Ciucci MR, et al. The science and practice of LSVT/LOUD: neural plasticity-principled approach to treating individuals with Parkinson disease and other neurological disorders. Semin Speech Lang 2006;27:283.

48. Turley R, Cohen S. Impact of voice and swallowing problems in the elderly. Otolaryngol Head Neck Surg 2009;140:33.

49. Roy N, Stemple J, Merrill RM, et al. Epidemiology of voice disorders in the elderly: preliminary findings. Laryngoscope 2007;117:628.

50. Golub JS, Chen PH, Otto KJ, et al. Prevalence of perceived dysphonia in a geriatric population. J Am Geriatr Soc 2006;54:1736.

51. Verdonck-de Leeuw IM, Mahieu HF. Vocal aging and the impact on daily life: a longitudinal study. J Voice 2004;18:193.

52. Woo P, Casper J, Colton R, et al. Dysphonia in the aging: physiology versus disease. Laryngoscope 1992;102:139.

53. Lundy DS, Silva C, Casiano RR, et al. Cause of hoarseness in elderly patients. Otolaryngol Head Neck Surg 1998;118:481.

54. Hoare TJ, Thomson HG, Proops DW. Detection of laryngeal cancer—the case for early specialist assessment. J R Soc Med 1993;86:390.

55. American Academy of Otolaryngology-Head and Neck Surgery. Fact sheet: about your voice. Available at: http://www.entnet.org/Healthinformation/aboutvoice.cfm. Accessed March 2, 2010.

56. Garrett CG, Ossoff RH. Hoarseness. Med Clin North Am 1999;83:115.

Otalgia

Ryan E. Neilan, MD, Peter S. Roland, MD*

KEYWORDS

- Primary otalgia • Secondary otalgia • Ear infection
- Temporomandibular joint

Otalgia, pain in the ear, can be a consequence of otologic disease (primary or otogenic otalgia), or can arise from pathologic processes and structures other than the ear (secondary or referred otalgia). In children, ear disease is far and away the most common cause of otalgia but in adults secondary or referred otalgia is more common.[1]

Sensory innervation of the ear is complex. Branches of the fifth, seventh, ninth, and tenth cranial nerve along with cervical nerves 1, 2, and 3 all contribute to sensation in the middle ear, external auditory canal, auricle, and peri-auricular tissues. Irritation of any portion of these cranial nerves can result in otalgia. The site of irritation can be quite remote from the ear itself. For example, otalgia can be the sole manifestation of myocardial ischemia (ie, an angina equivalent) because the vagus nerve provides sensory innervations for both structures.[2–4]

The characteristics of the pain symptoms may provide important clues as to the etiology. Pain associated with infection is usually continuous (although it may wax and wane in intensity) and is likely to become progressively severe over hours or days. Infection is unlikely to produce pain that lasts for a few hours then resolves completely, only to return days or weeks later for brief time intervals. Intermittent pain is much more likely to be associated, for example, with musculoskeletal conditions. Temporomandibular joint (TMJ) dysfunction and other myofascial pain dysfunction syndromes commonly present in this fashion. Overall duration of otalgia symptoms may help to differentiate chronic from acute processes. Other associated symptoms such as otorrhea, hearing loss, aural fullness, or vertigo may point to an otogenic source for otalgia complaints (primary otalgia). A history of fever, sore throat, reflux symptoms, hoarseness, sinusitis symptoms, or recent dental work suggests referred otalgia. Physical examination should include careful inspection of the pinna, post auricular area, external auditory canal, and tympanic membrane. A full head and neck examination should be carried out including inspection of nasal cavity, oral cavity, neck, and possibly the larynx. In most cases, the history and physical findings are sufficient to diagnose the cause of otalgia. However, tympanometry, audiometry, and magnetic resonance imaging (MRI) or computed tomography (CT) may be

Department of Otolaryngology-Head & Neck Surgery, UT Southwestern Medical Center at Dallas, 5323 Harry Hines Boulevard, Dallas, TX 75390-9035, USA
* Corresponding author.
E-mail address: peter.roland@utsouthwestern.edu

Med Clin N Am 94 (2010) 961–971
doi:10.1016/j.mcna.2010.05.004
0025-7125/10/$ – see front matter © 2010 Elsevier Inc. All rights reserved.

required to secure a diagnosis. In general, persistent or otherwise unexplained otalgia symptoms should prompt referral for further evaluation.

PRIMARY OTALGIA

The most common cause of primary otalgia is acute infectious ear disease. Chronic otologic infections, on the other hand, are rarely painful and consequently when ear pain is encountered in the presence of chronic suppurative otitis media, chronic tympanic membrane perforation, chronic external otitis, or cholesteatoma, another and different cause for the ear pain should be diligently sought. Chronic myringitis may be an exception to this rule.[5]

Disorders of the External Ear

Acute folliculitis is exquisitely painful. The disease is generally the result of a gram-positive infection initiated in an occluded hair follicle. As a consequence the condition is generally restricted to the lateral external auditory canal where hair is found. In effect it becomes a small abscess. Folliculitis is best treated with systemic antibiotics directed against gram-positive organisms including Staphylococcus aureus. Incision and drainage of these small abscesses is occasionally necessary to relieve pain and hasten resolution.

Acute Bacterial External Otitis

Acute bacterial otitis externa (AOE) is a subdermal infection of the external auditory canal (EAC) that results from the breakdown of the natural skin and cerumen protective barrier that normally prevents bacterial infection. AOE is commonly termed "swimmer's ear" but may be caused by any condition that removes the natural protective barrier, often in conjunction with elevated humidity and temperature. The slightly acidic pH of the normal EAC is an important protective feature in normal ears, and alkalinization of the canal is one important predisposing factor. Canal obstruction from hearing aids, cerumen impaction, the use of an ear plug, chronic seborrheic dermatitis, and trauma from scratching are also recognized predisposing factors.

The major symptoms include pain, aural fullness, itching, and hearing loss. On physical examination the EAC may be either intensely erythematous or very swollen. Edema may completely close the EAC, preventing visualization of the medial canal and tympanic membrane. A scant, milky exudate is common. Cellulitis may be seen extending away from ear into the soft tissues of the face or retro-auricular area. The ear may be extremely tender, and even slight traction on the pinna or touching the tragus will be very painful, which distinguishes AOE from otitis media. Typical pathogens include Pseudomonas aeruginosa, S aureus, and other gram-negative bacilli. Often the infection is polymicrobial. Fungal involvement is uncommon in the acute setting.

Treatment begins with thoroughly cleaning the EAC of debris and exudates. In uncomplicated cases of acute otitis externa, topical therapy is all that is required. Topical ear drops deliver a very high concentration of the antimicrobial (2000–3000 µg/mL) to the affected tissues and minimize exposure of bacteria to subtherapeutic concentrations of antimicrobials, as occurs with systemic therapy.[6] This reduces selection for resistant organisms. No topical antimicrobial has been shown to be superior to any other, but the addition of a steroid has been shown in some studies to hasten the elimination of pain.[7] Proper administration of drops is important to ensure adequate dose delivery. Drops should be applied with the patient lying down and the affected ear upwards. Drops should be placed to fill the canal, the patient should remain in this position for 3 to 5 minutes, and the canal should be left open to air in order to dry. The most common cause of failure of medical therapy results from inadequate delivery of topical antibiotics secondary to inadequate debridement or swelling of the EAC. If the infection has progressed to the point where there is significant edema of the canal, it may interfere with placement of drops; a wick should be placed to ensure that the drops are getting into the canal. Once inserted the drops are placed onto the wick. The patient is reexamined several days later and the wick removed. If the edema persists, a new wick should be inserted. The canal should be assessed every 3 to 4 days to determine the need for a wick until the canal is again patent. It is advised that drops be continued 7 days after cessation of symptoms to ensure resolution of infection. Oral analgesia is usually adequate for pain control, but narcotics are often necessary. When frequent dosing of an analgesic is required, administration at fixed intervals may be more effective than dosing as necessary. The addition of oral antibiotics to the treatment regimen is appropriate when cellulitis extends beyond the limits of the canal into surrounding soft tissues of the face or auricle. When patients have certain predisposing risk factors such as diabetes, human immunodeficiency virus (HIV), or other immune deficiencies, systemic antibiotics should be started at the outset of the infection.[8,9] At present the drug of choice is an oral fluoroquinolone. It should be remembered that oral fluoroquinolones are not approved for use in patients younger than 18 years because there is a risk of cartilage injury. There is no contraindication to the use of fluoroquinolone otic drops in pediatric patients. When symptoms have not resolved after 10 to 14 days of this treatment, it should be presumed that the patient has necrotizing external otitis.

Necrotizing Otitis Externa

Special concern is appropriate for diabetics, immunocompromised patients, HIV-positive patients, and the elderly with persistent symptoms (especially persistent pain) despite therapy. In this population the diagnosis of necrotizing otitis externa must be entertained. Necrotizing external otitis (sometimes called "malignant otitis externa") represents extension of the infection into the underlying bone and is a potentially fatal condition. Symptoms include persistent, deep-seated otalgia for more than 1 week, persistent purulent otorrhea with granulation tissue in the ear canal, and/or the development of lower cranial nerve palsy, most commonly facial paralysis. In patients with such persistent symptoms a technetium-99m bone scan and referral to an otolaryngologist is warranted. Rapid intervention is necessary because progression to death can be rapid.[5]

Cerumen Impaction

Cerumen impaction, if severe enough and especially if it is acute, can result in significant dull, achy pain. Painful cerumen impaction is sometimes a consequence of attempts to remove cerumen. Instrumentation can produce microtrauma, and cotton applicators can push cerumen further into the ear can and compact it more tightly.[9]

Keratosis Obturans

Individuals with a pathologic condition termed keratitis obturans may also experience ear pain as a consequence of an occluded EAC. Individuals with keratitis obturans, usually in their second or third decade, accumulate large amounts of desquamated epithelial debris in the medial portions of their canal. As desquamated epithelium accumulates, pressure increases and pain can result. These individuals frequently develop bony remodeling of the medial EAC caused by pressure. The medial canal becomes dilated, which further exacerbates the tendency of desquamated epithelial debris to become trapped and compressed. Pain is relieved by removal of the impacted desquamated keratin debris.

Neoplasms

Some neoplasms of the external canal are often very painful, and squamous cell carcinoma of the EAC is the most important example. Other neoplasms (neuromas, basal cell carcinoma, meningiomas) may or may not be painful depending on the structures involved. Pain is especially worrisome if accompanied by bleeding. Deep boring pain associated with granulation tissue in the EAC should raise the suspicion of neoplasm in all individuals, but especially in elderly persons. Cholesteatoma of the EAC may present with a very similar appearance, and can sometimes be confidently diagnosed on physical examination if keratinizing squamous epithelium can be seen invading directly into bone, but great caution should be exercised in order to eliminate the possibility of squamous cell carcinoma. A contrast-enhanced CT scan to establish the extent of temporal bone involvement and help rule out the possibility of neoplastic origin is useful, but does not replace the biopsy of abnormal tissue that is almost always necessary.

Perichondritis and Chondritis

Perichondritis and chondritis refer to inflammation of the perichondrium and cartilage, respectively. These conditions may develop from infections such as otitis externa or may be the result of trauma to the pinna. The condition typically presents with severe pain and itching. The affected area is erythematous and edematous, and may progress to involve adjacent areas. Eventually the skin in the affected region will begin to desquamate and the underlying cartilage can begin to weep. Cultures of the infected area should be taken, with *Pseudomonas* and *S aureus* being common pathogens. Initial management includes use of topical and oral antibiotics. Flouroquinolones are commonly selected because they are active against both gram-positive and gram-negative organisms. If infection becomes chronic, with continued weeping despite medical management, surgical debridement of affected cartilage is indicated.

Relapsing Polychondritis

Relapsing polychondritis is an uncommon autoimmune disease characterized by recurrent bouts of cartilage inflammation that eventually progress to fibrosis of the affected tissues. Other organs are often involved in the autoimmune process, and otic involvement is often bilateral. The auricle is most frequently affected and may be the sole site of involvement, with otalgia the only complaint. The auricle is erythematous, swollen, and tender. The condition may progress to hearing loss resulting from either canal edema or eustachian tube closure in up to one-half of patients.[10] The lobule is not involved because it lacks cartilage, which helps to distinguish relapsing polychondritis from cellulitis.[5] Clinical manifestations are episodic and can occasionally be associated with fevers, weight loss, erythema, edema, and elevation of erythrocyte sedimentation rate during acute episodes. Biopsy of the affected tissue will display cartilage necrosis, inflammation, and fibrosis. Of particular concern in these patients is that many will develop involvement of cartilaginous structures of the airway.[11,12] Symptoms such as dysphonia, shortness of breath, and stridor suggest airway involvement. Treatment involves use of oral corticosteroids and other immunomodulating drugs.

Disorders of the Middle Ear

Acute otitis media (AOM) is characterized by the presence of fluid in the middle ear space together with signs and symptoms of inflammation. AOM is most common in children and is usually the result of an acute bacterial infectious process. The organisms commonly recovered are *Streptococcus pneumoniae*, *Haemophilus influenzae*, and *Moraxella catarrhalis*. The pain associated with AOM may begin as a mild aching, often associated with decreased or "muffled" hearing. Pain increases in severity until effective therapy is implemented, spontaneous resolution begins, or the ear drum ruptures.

At its worst, the pain of AOM is described as severe, pulsating, aching pain centered over the ear canal. Rupture of the ear drum usually results in a sudden, marked decrease in pain and defervescence of fever. Although pain may be very severe, the ear is not tender, which serves to distinguish middle ear disease from conditions of the EAC. A majority of cases (about 80%) of AOM will resolve spontaneously and consequently, some physicians allow a day or two of observation before the institution of systemic antibiotic therapy. If after 24 to 48 hours symptoms and physical findings have not improved (or have worsened), antibiotic treatment is begun. However, even if antibiotic treatment is withheld, sufficient analgesics for adequate pain control must be provided.

Bullous myringitis, an acute bacterial infection involving the tympanic membrane, results in the formation of bullae or blebs that can be easily seen on the tympanic membrane using an otoscope. Bullous myringitis is especially painful, and is most common in children but occurs occasionally in adults. The bacterial causes of bullous myringitis are now regarded to be essentially the same as those that cause AOM. Puncturing the blebs on the tympanic membrane, while painful for a few seconds, can result in significant diminution of pain thereafter.

Barotrauma

Acute barotrauma, usually associated with flying or scuba diving, can be extremely painful.[3] Rapid development of negative pressure in the middle ear space causes rupture of vessels, which can produce submucosal bleeding and hematoma formation. Bleeding can also occur within the substance of the tympanic membrane itself. Negative pressure in the middle ear space can cause acute retraction of the tympanic membrane and can result in tympanic membrane rupture. Acute barotitis is often associated with barotrauma in the perinasal sinuses, which involves similar pathologic processes and also results in pain.

Mastoiditis

Acute mastoiditis is relatively rare with the widespread use of antibiotics, but is currently on the increase.[12] Mastoiditis generally develops from AOM and may develop despite previous antibiotic therapy. If an episode of AOM does not respond after 7 days of therapy, mastoiditis should be considered. Common symptoms include otalgia, postauricular pain, and fever. Otorrhea and hearing loss may also be present. There may be protrusion of the pinna and postauricular erythema. Postauricular induration and fluctuance may represent an underlying subperiosteal abscess. External otitis can produce physical findings similar to mastoiditis if canal inflammation is sufficiently severe to involve postauricular tissues. Undiagnosed mastoiditis can lead to severe complications such as facial paralysis, labyrinthitis, extradural abscess, meningitis, brain abscess, sigmoid sinus thrombophlebitis, and otitic hydrocephalus. Because the diagnosis depends on changes in bony anatomy of the mastoid air cell system, CT is the preferred imaging modality; MRI is useful if intracranial complications are suspected. The diagnosis is radiographic. A CT scan will show bony destruction of the mastoid air cells with coalescence of air cells into a single cavity. Fluid filling intact mastoid air cells does not constitute mastoiditis.

The initial treatment of mastoiditis is intravenous antibiotic therapy. Typical empiric coverage includes vancomycin plus ceftriaxone to be followed by culture-specific therapy if otorrhea is present. Although some cases may be treated by hospitalization and intravenous antibiotics alone, other cases, particularly those with any evidence of intracranial progression, need a mastoidectomy with myringotomy. Management of these situations is best left to the otologic surgeon.

Previous Ear Surgery

Chronic pain can follow surgical procedures of the ear and mastoid. The precise etiology is often unclear and treatment can be difficult. Postauricular pain following mastoidectomy is the most common presentation. The edges of the mastoid cavity are tender to palpation, and one can often palpate an irregular margin of the cavity due to osteoneogenesis. As with other forms of postsurgical ear pain, treatment usually consists of nonsteroidal anti-inflammatory agents. Local injections of anesthetic and/or steroids are employed occasionally.

SECONDARY OTALGIA

Secondary or referred otalgia is suggested when the physical examination of the ear is entirely normal but pain is experienced as arising in the ear or peri-auricular tissues. It is important to recognize that the severity of pain does not correlate with the gravity of its underlying cause: very severe pain can, for example, be a consequence of viral pharyngitis whereas a mild, dull aching can represent a carcinoma of the larynx. Charlett and Coatesworth[13] indicate that lesions of the anterior tongue and floor of the mouth usually refer pain to the ear canal or concha, whereas pathology involving the lateral base of tongue, tonsil, or lower two-thirds of the nasopharynx is felt as intense pain deep in the ear.

Oro-Maxillofacial Etiologies

Sinusitis

The maxillary and ethmoid sinuses are innervated by the second division of the fifth cranial nerve and, therefore, can be a source of referred otalgia. Acute, and less commonly chronic, sinusitis can generate dull, aching ear pain that waxes and wanes in severity. Pain and tenderness of the maxillary molars is common. Nasal obstruction (a "stuffy" nose) is the most common symptom but mucopurulent rhinorhea, anosmia, and postnasal drip are frequently present. Fever, malaise, and other constitutional symptoms are present only when the process is acute. Physical examination in acute disease will demonstrate inflamed, engorged nasal mucosa, nasal obstruction, and mucopurulent nasal drainage. Physical findings in chronic sinusitis are highly variable, but nasal obstruction and inflamed mucosa are often present. Treatment of acute disease is with systemic antibiotics, decongestants, nasal saline sprays or irrigations, and analgesics. The management of chronic disease is complex and variable, often including topical nasal steroids, nasal irrigations, and episodic use of antibiotics (both topical and systemic).

Dental structures are innervated by the fifth cranial nerve, and dental disorders are common causes of referred pain to the ear. Impacted wisdom teeth, poorly fitting dentures, and peri-apical abscesses are common causes of referred ear pain.[14]

A history of dental disease should be sought, and the oropharynx and dentition carefully inspected. Occasionally, gentle percussion of each tooth individually using a tongue blade will cause pain and will identify the involved tooth. Gingiva may be swollen, erythematous, edematous, and tender. If tooth decay extends through dentine into the tooth pulp, pain is often poorly localized and commonly radiates to the cheek and ear.[10] Oral ulcers, including aphthous ulcers, can result in ear pain, especially if they are located in the posterior tongue or peri-tonsillar area.

Temporomandibular joint disorders

TMJ-related disorders were the cause of ear pain in about 25% of subjects with referred otalgia in one large study.[15] TMJ disorders are a collection of musculoskeletal disorders affecting the joint, the muscles of mastication, or both. Approximately 65% of patients with TMJ disorders complain of otalgia.[13,16] Pain can arise as a consequence of intrinsic joint disease or as a consequence of spasm in the muscles of mastication (temporalis, masseter, internal and external pterygoids). Bruxism (teeth grinding), teeth clenching while sleeping, malocclusion (especially overbite), previous maxillofacial trauma, and emotional stress are all thought to be predisposing factors. Symptoms of intrinsic joint disease include popping and clicking with mouth opening, displacement of the disc, which locks the jaw open, and a palpable lurching of the condyle when the mouth is opened and closed. The presence of crepitus on examination does not always imply TMJ as the cause of the patient's otalgia, as can be found on examination of normal patients.[5] Other disorders involving the joint itself include synovitis, disc dislocation, and osteoarthritis. Pain varies in intensity but can be very severe. It is usually epicentered over the joint or EAC. When nocturnal bruxism or nocturnal teeth clenching is the origin, pain is often most severe in the morning on awakening and improves during the course of the day. The joint is often tender to palpation. The joint itself should be palpated during active motion to assess for pain. TMJ disorders may also be associated with symptoms of aural fullness, tinnitus, and vertigo.[17,18] Myofascial pain has been implicated as a common cause of the otalgia component in TMJ syndromes. This condition is characterized by a regional dull pain of moderate intensity that is aggravated by mastication secondary to reflex splinting of the muscle groups. Spasm of the muscles of mastication may occur together with intrinsic joint disease or with an entirely normal joint. Examination will detect tenderness in one or more of the muscles of mastication, and very tender" trigger points" may be present. The joint itself, however, is usually nontender unless there is associated intrinsic joint disease. In the absence of intrinsic joint disease pain can be variable and diffuse; it can be retro-auricular, felt "deep in the ear," or temporal. The medial pterygoid muscle can refer pain to behind and below the TMJ as well as deep in the ear, and may be associated with aural fullness. The lateral pterygoid refers pain deep into the TMJ and is often the source of referred pain, and can be mistaken for arthritis of the joint itself. When the temporalis muscle is prominently involved, recurrent temporal headache is a common complaint. Intraoral palpation of the pterygoid muscles should be performed to evaluate for spasm.

The mainstay of therapy involves resting the joint and muscles by eating a soft diet, avoiding chewing gum, and the application of heat. Non steroidal anti-inflammatory agents are the most common medication used, though refractory cases sometimes require low-dose tricyclic antidepressants or a short course of oral steroids. Oral splints (mouth guards) have been used extensively in the treatment of TMJ syndrome, although their efficacy remains controversial and long-term complications of use can require orthodontics or surgery for correction.[19] At present, splints should only be used for short-term therapy and not as the sole therapy. Surgery is reserved for those few cases where medical management is not effective in improving symptoms. Surgery is appropriate for those cases where a structural defect in the joint can be identified by imaging or arthroscopy. Care must be taken to consider other causes such as myofascial pain before attempting surgery. Less invasive procedures such as arthroscopy are usually attempted before more open invasive procedures.

Cervical disease

A variety of conditions involving the neck can produce referred otalgia. Inflammatory thyroiditis can produce referred ear pain as can simple adenopathy, especially if it is of inflammatory origin. Carotidenia (inflammation of the carotid sheath) is associated principally with dysphagia and odynophagia as well as local carotid tenderness, but inflammation produced by reflux can produce inflammation in the larynx, pharynx, and at the origin of the facial tube. Such reflux can, as part of the overall symptom complex, include referred pain to one or both ears. Primary symptoms will depend on which portion of the upper aerodigestive tract and which ear has been most irritated; hoarseness and sinusitis have both been attributed to laryngotracheal reflux and, in children, it is believed to be one cause of chronic middle ear effusion and AOM.[15,18]

Myofascial pain syndromes

Myofascial pain dysfunction syndromes arise when muscles develop trigger points, tight bands, and shortening.[10] It commonly involves the muscles of mastication, the lateral cervical, posterior cervical, and shoulder muscles, and is commonly associated with degenerative cervical spine disease. In the study by Jaber and colleagues[15] of 123 patients with referred otalgia, cervical spine etiologies were the most common cause of referred ear pain, accounting for more than 35% of cases. The prevalence of cervical myofascial pain dysfunction syndrome has been estimated to be 3.6% to 7.0% of the population.[10] Ear pain, often described as felt "deep in the ear," aural fullness, and subjective hearing loss (not verified on objective testing) are common symptoms. Pain referral patterns from various muscle groups to the ear and peri-auricular area have been well worked out and are repeatable.[19,20] The presence of pain is often variable, and pain can disappear and reemerge over fairly short intervals. Pain intensity varies as well, but the pain can be severe. A history of neck pain can be elicited in the majority of patients with cervically related myofascial pain dysfunction syndrome. The diagnosis depends on identifying the muscle pathology, but is supported by the presence of findings of degenerative upper cervical spine disease on radiographic imaging (usually MRI), which is present in the great majority of cases.[15] Physical examination focuses on careful inspection of the muscles of mastication, and cervical and shoulder musculature. Localized trigger points, which are tender or can reproduce pain, are identified by palpation. One trigger point in the upper trapezius fibers has been shown to refer pain up the posterior aspect of the neck to the mastoid and posterior auricular area.[20] Vertigo and disequilibrium are sometimes associated with myofascial pain dysfunction syndromes.[10] Treatment includes nonsteroidal anti-inflammatory agents and physical therapy. Physical therapy may include ice, heat massage, myofascial release, and range-of-motion exercises. In severe cases trigger points are treated with injection of local anesthetic.

Facial paralysis

Both acute cryptogenic facial paralysis (Bell palsy) and facial paralysis associated with herpes zoster oticus (Ramsey-Hunt syndrome) are associated with pain. The pain is less severe with Bell palsy, and usually consists of 1 to 3 days of achy retro-auricular-mastoid pain often starting a day or two before the onset of facial weakness.

The pain rarely persists more than 24 to 36 hours after the onset of facial paralysis. Acute viral infection of the facial nerve is believed to be the cause of Bell palsy, and spontaneous recovery is the rule. However, 15% or more of patients fail to recover acceptable facial function following episodes of Bell palsy, and consequently most clinicians treat Bell palsy with a short course of high-dose systemic steroids and 7 to 10 days of antiviral medication.[21,22]

Ramsey-Hunt syndrome is a more severe viral infection and involves the geniculate ganglion. Ramsey-Hunt syndrome is frequently accompanied by dysfunction of cranial nerves VII and VIII: a significant balance disturbance and sensorineural hearing loss often accompany the facial paralysis. Pain with Ramsey-Hunt syndrome can be severe and can persist for months after the onset of facial weakness. The pain alone can make this a debilitating disease, and oral narcotic analgesic agents are frequently required in a short and intermediate period. Indeed, one way of distinguishing Ramsey-Hunt syndrome from Bell palsy is by the severity of pain associated with the facial paralysis. The most important diagnostic feature, however, is the appearance of vesicles in the EAC, on the tympanic membrane or around the auricle. These vesicles are typical herpetic lesions, which may appear as early as a week before the onset of facial paralysis or may occur days after the onset of facial paralysis. The simultaneous occurrence of acute rapid onset of facial paralysis and vesicular lesions involving the EAC is virtually pathoneumonic for herpes zoster oticus. A short regimen of high-dose steroids is believed to make a significant difference in outcome when combined with high-dose antivirals. Because of their very much better absorption and higher blood levels, either valcyclovir or famcyclovir are preferred to oral acyclovir. If acyclovir is used, intravenous administration is preferable in order to achieve adequate blood levels.

Disorders of the Aerodigestive Tract

Because sensation to the pharynx and the larynx is provided by cranial nerves 9 and 10, pathology in the hypopharynx and larynx are common causes of referred otalgia. Referred pain is not uncommonly perceived to be of greater intensity and severity than the pain at the primary site of pathology. Any lesion of the posterior or lateral oropharynx can produce referred otalgia including ulcers, inflammatory conditions, and benign or malignant neoplasms. Pharyngitis and tonsillitis frequently feature ear pain as an associated symptom. Otalgia is frequent following tonsillectomy. Calcification of the styloid ligament leading to elongation of the styloid process (Eagle syndrome) is an uncommon cause of referred otalgia. An elongated styloid process can be palpated manually in the tonsillar fossa and is generally visible on radiographs. Local pain in the tonsillar fossa along with referred pain to the ipsilateral ear is exacerbated by swallowing. Most patients have had a previous tonsillectomy. Pain is relieved with resection of the elongated styloid.

Supraglottic laryngitis ("epiglottis") typically has severe otalgia as an associated symptom. This condition is characterized by severe pharyngitis, hoarseness, pain on swallowing, and fever. In children especially, supraglottic edema can lead to life-threatening upper airway obstruction. Arytenoid arthritis, similarly, can produce referred ear pain associated with hoarseness. Arytenoid movement exacerbates pain and therefore pain is worse on speaking, coughing, or swallowing.

Otalgia may be the only or most prominent symptom of a neoplasm. Unexplained otalgia, especially in an adult, requires complete evaluation of the entire pharynx including the nasopharynx and the larynx, to identify or rule out an occult neoplasm. Neoplastic disease should be suspected especially if there are associated symptoms of weight loss, odynophagia, dysphagia, or hoarseness. Risk factors include smoking, high alcohol intake, and age older than 50 years. Evaluation should include careful visual examination of the pharynx, palpation of the base of the tongue, direct and/or indirect evaluation of the hypopharynx and the larynx, careful palpation of the neck and, if physical examination fails to reveal the origin, complete radiographic examination of the upper aerodigestive tract. If an initial evaluation fails to identify the cause of otalgia and the otalgia persists, physical and radiologic examination needs to be repeated at appropriate intervals until the cause is identified or the otalgia resolves.

SUMMARY

Otalgia is a common complaint with diverse causes. While many causes are otologic in nature, one must remember that referred pain from other areas of the head and neck are common. This situation is attributed to the complex innervation of structures in this area by the fifth, seventh, ninth, and tenth cranial nerves. A comprehensive history and physical examination are essential in identifying these other potential causes. Identification of the disease process can ensure quick initiation of treatment and referral if necessary for further or definitive care. In most instances referral to an otolaryngologist is appropriate, but in cases involving TMJ or otalgia thought to be from an odontogenic source, referral to an oral surgeon may be more appropriate. Otalgia can be the only presenting symptom of several serious conditions, and its etiology should be fully explored. Unfortunately, its workup is complex and no simple algorithm exists. The causes of otalgia outlined here represent the most common ones, and should always be considered.

REFERENCES

1. Majumdar S, Wu K, Bateman ND, et al. Diagnosis and management of otalgia in children. Arch Dis Child Educ Pract Ed 2009;94:33–6.
2. Yanagisawa K, Kveton JF. Referred otalgia. Am J Otolaryngol 1992;136:323–7.
3. Mirza S, Richardson H. Otic barotraumas from air travel. J Laryngol Otol 2005; 119:366–70.
4. Ely JW, Hansen MR, Clark EC. Diagnosis of ear pain. Am Fam Physician 2008; 775:621–8.
5. Shah RK, Blevins NH. Otalgia. Otolaryngol Clin North Am 2003;36:1137–51.
6. Rosenfeld RM, Singer M, Wasserman JM, Stinnett SS. Systematic review of topical antimicrobial therapy for acute otitis externa [review]. Otolaryngol Head Neck Surg 2006;134(Suppl 4):S24–48.
7. Rosenfeld RM, Brown L, Cannon CR, et al. Clinical practice guideline: acute otitis externa. Otolaryngol Head Neck Surg 2006;134(Suppl 4):S4–23.
8. Roland PS. External otitis: a challenge in management. Curr Infect Dis Rep 2000; 2(2):160–7.
9. Roland PS, Smith TL, Schwartz SR, et al. Clinical practice guideline: cerumen impaction. Otolaryngol Head Neck Surg 2008;139:S1–21.
10. Teachey WS. Otolaryngic myofascial pain syndromes. Curr Pain Headache Rep 2004;8(6):457–62.
11. Trentham D, Le C. Relapsing polychondritis. Ann Intern Med 1998;129:114–22.
12. Geva A, Oestreicher-Kedem Y, Fishman G, et al. Conservative management of acute mastoiditis in children. Int J Pediatr Otorhinolaryngol 2008;72(5):629–34.
13. Charlett SD, Coatesworth AP. Referred otalgia: a structured approach to diagnosis and treatment. Int J Clin Pract 2007;61(6):1015–21.
14. Kreisberg MK, Turner J. Dental causes of referred otalgia. Ear Nose Throat J 1987;66:398–408.

15. Jaber J, Leonetti J, Lawrason A, et al. Cervical spine causes for referred otalgia. Otolaryngol Head Neck Surg 2008;138(4):479–85.
16. Kim DS, Cheang P, Dover S, et al. Dental otalgia. J Laryngol Otol 2007;121: 1129–34.
17. Cooper BC, Cooper DI. Recognizing otolaryngologic symptoms in patients with temporamandibular joint symptoms. Cranio 1993;11:260–7.
18. Ulualp SO, Toohill RJ, Shaker R. Pharyngeal acid reflux in patients with single and multiple otolaryngologic disorders. Otolaryngol Head Neck Surg 1999;121(6): 725–30.
19. Klasser GD, Greene CS. Oral appliances in the management of temporomandibular disorders. Oral Surg Oral Med Oral Pathol Oral Radiol Endod 2009;107(2): 212–23.
20. Simons DG, Travel JG, Simons LS. Myofascial pain and dysfunction: the trigger point manual. In: The upper half of body, vol. 1. 2nd edition. Lippincott, Williams & Wilkins; 1999. p. 278–81, 308–11, 365–9, 379–83.
21. Quant EC, Jeste SS, Muni RH, et al. The benefits of steroids versus steroids plus antivirals for treatment of Bell's palsy: a meta-analysis [review]. BMJ 2009;339: b3354.
22. Muecke M, Amedee RG. Herpes zoster oticus: diagnosis and management. J La State Med Soc 1993;145(8):333–5.

Hearing Loss

Brandon Isaacson, MD

KEYWORDS
- Hearing loss • Hearing examinations
- Diagnosis and treatment • Ear

Hearing loss is one of the most common sensory impairments and affects almost 10% of the adult population. The percentage of adults with hearing loss markedly increases with advancing age. Continuing advances in medical care will result in further prolongation of life expectancy and will likely increase the number of individuals with hearing loss.[1,2]

ANATOMY

The perception of sound requires a complex series of structures, including the external auditory canal, tympanic membrane, ossicles (malleus, incus, and stapes), cochlea, eighth cranial nerve, brainstem auditory pathways, and the auditory cortex. Disease affecting any one of these structures ultimately results in hearing loss (**Fig. 1**).[3]

PHYSIOLOGY

A detailed description of the physiology of sound perception is beyond the scope of this article and only a basic description is provided. Sound is transmitted through the external auditory canal and contacts the tympanic membrane, which has a larger surface area than the stapes footplate. This area mismatch provides most impedance matching between the sound wave in environmental air and the inner ear fluids. Compression and rarefaction of the inner ear fluids by the stapes footplate are further enhanced by the lever action of the malleus and incus. Displacement of the inner ear fluids results in depolarization of the hair cells in the organ of Corti. The base of the depolarized hair cell then activates the cochlear division of the eighth cranial nerve via synaptic transmission. The action potential from the eighth cranial nerve ultimately gets processed via the auditory brainstem and cortex and results in the perception of sound.[3]

CATEGORIES OF HEARING LOSS

Hearing loss is typically categorized as conductive, sensorineural, or mixed conductive and sensorineural. Conductive hearing loss results when sound is unable to

---

Department of Otolaryngology - Head and Neck Surgery, UT - Southwestern Medical Center, 5323 Harry Hines Boulevard, Dallas, TX 75390-9035, USA
E-mail address: brandon.isaacson@utsouthwestern.edu

Med Clin N Am 94 (2010) 973–988
doi:10.1016/j.mcna.2010.05.003
0025-7125/10/$ – see front matter © 2010 Elsevier Inc. All rights reserved.

disease, labyrinthitis, neoplasm involving or compressing the eighth cranial nerve, brainstem ischemia/infarct, perilymph fistula). Ear pain (otalgia) occurring concurrently with hearing loss often indicates disease of the ear canal or middle ear (ear canal or middle ear neoplasm, otitis externa, otitis media, trauma). Ear fullness or pressure may be seen in conditions such as Meniere disease, otitis media, otitis externa, eighth nerve neoplasm, and middle ear or ear canal neoplasm.

PHYSICAL EXAMINATION
Otoscopy

A handheld otoscope can be used to determine the status of the ear canal, tympanic membrane, the middle ear, and in some cases the ossicular chain. A pneumatic bulb attachment allows the examiner to assess tympanic membrane mobility.

Tuning Fork Examination

Tuning forks provide a simple, yet powerful means to examine a patient's hearing. The 512-Hz tuning fork is the most commonly used for the Weber and Rinne tests. The Weber test requires the examiner to place the tuning fork on the midline forehead and ask the patient in which ear they hear the sound. If the hearing is symmetric the patient is not able to discern which side is louder. If unilateral SNHL is present the patient hears the sound in the better-hearing ear. With a unilateral conductive loss the patient hears the sound in the affected ear. The Rinne test requires the examiner to place the tuning fork behind the patient's ear until the patient can no longer hear the sound and then the tuning fork is placed lateral to the external ear. If the sound is louder behind the ear a conductive hearing loss is present, whereas if the sound is louder lateral to the ear the hearing is normal or SNHL is present (**Fig. 2**; **Table 1**).[6]

DIFFERENTIAL DIAGNOSIS
Diagnostics

Audiogram
The audiogram is most commonly performed by an audiologist or occasionally an otolaryngologist (**Table 2**). The clinician should consider obtaining an audiogram in any patient presenting with unilateral or bilateral hearing loss. The audiogram is a subjective and objective test of auditory function and has several components. Audiograms are conducted in a soundproof booth to limit the effect of background noise. Pure tone audiometry is a subjective assessment of hearing that involves the presentation of various frequencies at various sound levels (volume). Pure tone testing relies on the subject responding when they hear the pure tone presented. Speech testing is another subjective method of auditory assessment, in which the subject is presented with a list of words and is asked to repeat these words. The percentage of correct words repeated results in a speech discrimination score, which is often decreased with a retrocochlear lesion (eg, acoustic neuroma, meningioma). Tympanometry is an objective test that assesses the mobility of the tympanic membrane and the pressure status of the middle ear. Tympanometry can identify the presence of negative middle ear pressure, middle ear effusion, and increased or decreased tympanic membrane mobility.[4]

MRI
MRI provides little to no information on the osseous detail, but is excellent at distinguishing the various soft-tissue conditions affecting the temporal bone. MRI is the study of choice for patients with unilateral or asymmetric SNHL.[7]

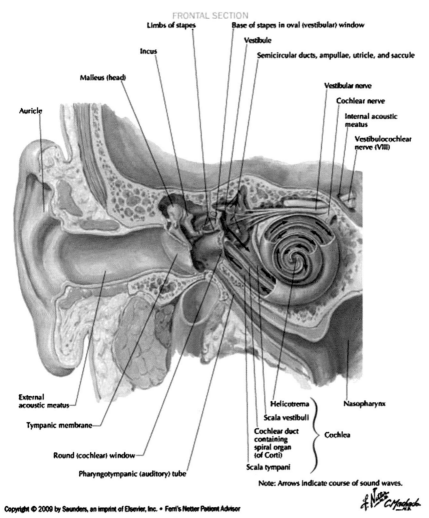

FRONTAL SECTION

Limbs of stapes   Base of stapes in oval (vestibular) window

Vestibule

Incus

Semicircular ducts, ampullae, utricle, and saccule

Malleus (head)

Vestibular nerve

Auricle

Cochlear nerve

Internal acoustic meatus

Vestibulocochlear nerve (VIII)

External acoustic meatus

Helicotrema

Nasopharynx

Scala vestibuli

Tympanic membrane

Cochlear duct containing spiral organ (of Corti)

Cochlea

Round (cochlear) window

Scala tympani

Pharyngotympanic (auditory) tube

Note: Arrows indicate course of sound waves.

Fig. 2. Anatomy of the external, middle, and inner ear (Reprinted from Netter Anatomy Illustration Collection, © Elsevier Inc. All Rights Reserved.).

Temporal bone computed tomography

Temporal bone computed tomography (CT) provides the clinician with intricate details of the osteology of the temporal bone. This modality easily identifies bone erosion involving the mastoid, facial nerve canal, inner ear, and ossicles. Temporal bone CT can also identify abnormal soft tissue within the middle ear or mastoid but does not identify what the soft tissue represents. For instance, a temporal bone CT does not allow the clinician to distinguish a middle ear effusion from a cholesteatoma or a neoplasm.[8]

Presbycusis

The most common cause of hearing loss is age-related degeneration of the inner ear, otherwise known as presbycusis. Fifty percent of individuals older than 75 years are affected with hearing loss, with the most common cause being presbycusis. Age-related hearing loss is sensorineural and typically affects the high frequencies first and

Table 3
NIOSH limits of noise exposure in the workplace	
Hours Per Day	Sound Levels (dB)
16	85
8	90
6	92
4	95
2	100
1	105
0.5	110
0.25	115

education, selection and use of hearing protection devices, and periodic assessments of hearing to prevent occupational noise-induced hearing loss.[13]

Sudden SNHL

Sudden SNHL is considered an otologic emergency. Patients should be referred for audiometric testing as soon as possible. Sudden SNHL is almost always unilateral and the hearing loss typically occurs immediately. Patients often describe a plugged sensation in the affected ear and also describe an abnormal sound perception (tinnitus). Acute room-spinning vertigo can also occur, which indicates a pathologic process affecting the cochlea and the vestibular system, otherwise known as labyrinthitis. The prevailing theory on the pathophysiology of sudden SNHL is an inflammatory/infectious event within the inner ear. The other common pathologic process is a vascular insult to the inner ear.[14]

MRI to assess the inner ear and eighth nerve is recommended for all patients presenting with sudden SNHL. Although most of these studies are normal, occasionally MRI reveals pathologic conditions such as an acoustic neuroma, meningioma, or inner ear hemorrhage, which can present as sudden SNHL. Most studies advocate the use of a 10- to 14-day course of oral corticosteroids. The addition of antivirals has not been supported by the most recent studies. The addition of intratympanic steroids in combination with oral steroids, as sole treatment, or as salvage therapy for those patients who have not responded to oral therapy, has been supported by recent studies.[15]

Meniere disease

Meniere disease is an idiopathic inner ear disorder characterized by fluctuating SNHL, episodic vertigo, tinnitus, and ear fullness or pressure. The pathophysiology of Meniere disease has not been completely elucidated. Excessive endolymph production from the stria vascularis or reduced endolymph resorption in the endolymphatic sac are the more common prevailing theories on the pathogenesis of Meniere disease.[16] The incidence of Meniere disease is approximately 40 per 100,000, with a peak onset between 40 and 60 years of age.[17] Meniere disease typically presents with unilateral auditory symptoms but can affect the contralateral ear at some point in up to 47% of patients.[18] Vertigo from Meniere disease can last from minutes to hours. The initial onset of Meniere disease is characterized by fluctuating, low-frequency SNHL. Most patients progress to moderate to severe SNHL within the first several years after the onset of symptoms.[19] Initial management with a low-sodium diet (<2000 mg per day) and a diuretic (combination hydrochlorothiazide and triamterene) has been shown to reduce the severity and frequency of vertigo but has no affect on hearing loss or tinnitus.[20] The use of betahistine, a capillary vasodilator, has been shown to reduce vertigo and improve the cochlear symptoms (hearing loss, tinnitus) in patients with Meniere disease.[21] Endolymphatic sac surgery, intratympanic gentamicin, labyrinthectomy, and vestibular neurectomy are potential treatment options for the 10% to 20% of patients who fail medical therapy.[22–24] Patients may benefit from amplification with a hearing aid or a cochlear implant, depending on the extent of the hearing loss.[25]

Acoustic neuroma

Acoustic neuroma, more appropriately termed vestibular schwannoma, is a slow-growing, benign neoplasm arising off the vestibular portion of the eighth cranial nerve. Acoustic neuromas comprise 6% of all intracranial tumors, with an estimated population incidence of 10 per million per year.[26,27] Most vestibular schwannomas are sporadic and unilateral, with the mean age of patients at presentation being 50 years old.[28] Approximately 5% of patients, who typically are diagnosed at a younger age, present with bilateral tumors consistent with diagnosis of neurofibromatosis type 2.[29] Ninety-five percent of patients with vestibular schwannoma present with unilateral or asymmetric SNHL. The hearing loss associated with vestibular schwannomas can vary from mild to profound. Approximately 26% of patients with vestibular schwannoma present with a sudden hearing loss.[30] Other common presenting symptoms include: tinnitus (70%), vertigo (19%), disequilibrium (70%), facial numbness (50%), headache (20%–40%), and facial twitching (10%).[28,30]

MRI with gadolinium is the study of choice to identify a vestibular schwannoma and can identify tumors as small as 1 mm. These tumors appear isointense on T1-weighted images, hypointense on T2-weighted images, and vividly enhance with gadolinium. Most vestibular schwannomas are centered in the internal auditory canal and can have variable extension into the cerebellopontine angle.[31] Observation with serial MRI examinations has become a well-accepted and in many cases the preferred management option in patients with small to medium-sized vestibular schwannomas. Hearing in patients with vestibular schwannomas can remain stable for many years without any intervention other than serial MRI.[32] Stereotactic radiation (Gamma Knife [Elekta, Stockholm, Sweden], Cyberknife [Accuray, Sunnyvale, CA, USA], Novalis [Brainlab, Westchester, IL, USA]) is a nonsurgical option that delivers highly conformal radiation to a lesion and that limits the dose to the surrounding structures. Hearing preservation rates with stereotactic radiation have significantly improved with the lower prescription doses that have been used since the 1990s.[33] In patients with larger tumors (>2 cm), stereotactic radiation offers the only realistic option for hearing preservation. Disadvantages of stereotactic radiation include potential for continued tumor enlargement, and less than ideal long-term hearing preservation, potential for radiation-induced neoplasia, need for repeat MRI examinations, and less than ideal facial nerve outcomes with microsurgery with tumors that show progressive enlargement.[34–36] Microsurgical excision of vestibular schwannomas in most cases allows for complete removal of the tumor. Tumors that are less than 1.8 cm in maximum diameter are potential candidates for hearing preservation surgery. Successful long-term hearing preservation is a distinct advantage of microsurgery in patients who have serviceable hearing.[37] Disadvantages of microsurgery include risk of temporary or permanent facial nerve paralysis, immediate risk of hearing loss, prolonged disequilibrium, stroke, death, risk of cerebrospinal fluid leak, or meningitis.[38]

Ototoxicity

Numerous topical and systemic compounds have the potential for ototoxicity. The most common agents responsible for ototoxicity are the aminoglycosides. Neomycin, kanamycin, dihydrostreptomycin, and amikacin are preferentially toxic to the cochlea, whereas tobramycin, gentamicin, and streptomycin are toxic to the vestibular system. The incidence of ototoxicity increases in the setting of renal failure because these medications are exclusively eliminated by the kidney. Aminoglycoside otoxicity is more associated with total dose than serum levels, thus peak and trough levels are not reliable predictors of this potentially devastating complication. Other potential risk factors associated with aminoglycoside ototoxicity include age greater than 60 years, preexisting SNHL, renal insufficiency, concurrent administration of other ototoxic agents, concurrent noise exposure, extended duration of therapy, and serum drug levels. There is also a known mitochondrial mutation that significantly increases the risk of aminoglycoside ototoxicity. The physician should consider ceasing an ototoxic medication when a patient reports new-onset hearing loss or tinnitus. There are a number of clinical and basic science reports that show the ototoxic effects of platinum-based chemotherapy agents (cisplatin, carboplatin). Other commonly known ototoxic medications include aspirin, macrolide antibiotics, and loop diuretics, quinine, and salicylates.[39,40]

Congenital hearing loss
Most congenital hearing loss in developed countries is discovered before hospital discharge because of the widespread implementation of newborn hearing screening programs. There are a plethora of causes for congenital SNHL. Prenatal viral infections, including cytomegalovirus, rubella, rubeola, herpes, and mumps, all have the potential to cause significant SNHL. Other causes of congenital hearing loss include syphilis and toxoplasmosis.[41,42]

There are numerous genetic causes of SNHL. Genetic hearing loss is typically divided into syndromic, nonsyndromic, autosomal recessive, autosomal dominant, mitochondrial, and X-linked. Most genetic hearing loss is nonsyndromic and autosomal recessive. The most common cause of genetic hearing loss is related to mutations in the GJB2 gene, which codes for connexin 26. Genetic testing for connexin 26 mutations is widely available.[43]

TRAUMA

Trauma that is not caused by excessive noise exposure most commonly occurs in association with a head injury. Motor vehicle accidents, assault, and other common causes of head trauma can result in various degrees of hearing loss depending on the severity of the injury. Hearing loss from trauma can be conductive, sensorineural, or mixed conductive-sensorineural. The mechanism for conductive hearing loss can be from a tympanic membrane perforation, or even disarticulation or fracture of the ossicles, which commonly occurs with temporal bone fractures. Hemorrhage into the middle ear space from trauma (hemotympanum) typically results in a conductive hearing loss that resolves with time. A temporal bone fracture that traverses the inner ear or internal auditory canal usually results in permanent severe to profound SNHL. Penetrating injuries to the temporal bone particularly from guns often result in permanent profound SNHL from direct injury or a blast injury to the inner ear.[44]

OTITIS MEDIA

Otitis media is one of the most common infections in childhood. The presence of fluid (pus, serous fluid) results in a conductive hearing loss because the mobility of the tympanic membrane and ossicles is limited. Otoscopy typically reveals a dull tympanic membrane with a diminished or absent light reflex. Air-fluid levels, air bubbles, or a bulging tympanic membrane with a yellow effusion may also be seen with the oto-scope. The conductive hearing loss resulting from otitis media almost always completely recovers once the middle ear fluid resolves. Middle ear effusion related to otitis media almost typically resolves within 3 months. Conductive hearing loss resulting from a prolonged middle ear effusion can be alleviated with a myringotomy and aspiration of the fluid or placement of a pressure equalization tube.[45]

OTITIS EXTERNA

Edema of the external auditory canal skin from otitis externa can result in significant obstructing edema of the external auditory canal. If the canal is almost or completely obstructed with edematous skin with or without squamous debris a significant conductive hearing loss can occur. Severe pain and tenderness with manipulation of the auricle are characteristic features of otitis externa, along with yellow-to-white debris. The conductive hearing loss resulting from otitis externa typically resolves in a matter of days once the debris are removed and topical combined steroid antibiotic drops are initiated. Placement of an expandable ear wick so topical drops can access the more medial aspect of the external auditory canal is used in cases with edema-related obstruction of the external auditory canal.[46] Chronic otitis externa can result in fibrosis of the medial ear canal skin, which can eventually obstruct the entire lumen of the external auditory canal, resulting in a significant conductive hearing loss.[47]

CERUMEN

Cerumen impaction is one of the most common causes of conductive hearing loss. Cerumen is a combination of devitalized squamous epithelium and sebaceous secre-tions. The cerumen typically lateralizes to the external meatus via epithelial migration. In some populations (eg, elderly or mentally impaired patients), this migration process is impaired and results in a cerumen impaction. Self-cleaning with cotton swabs or other items can often displace the cerumen more medially in the ear canal, further exacerbating the problem. A recent multispecialty guideline was released that discusses the indications and management options for cerumen impaction. Removal is recommended in impactions that result in hearing loss or limit a complete view of the medial aspect of the external auditory canal and tympanic membrane. Otomicroscopy with mechanical removal of the cerumen or ear canal irrigations are the preferred management options for cerumen impactions. There is now enough evidence to suggest that ear candling has no role in the management of cerumen and can be harmful in some cases. Patients who develop more frequent cerumen impactions can self-irrigate or use mineral oil on a regular basis to prevent recurrence.[48]

TYMPANIC MEMBRANE PERFORATION

Tympanic membrane perforations are typically associated with varying degrees of conductive hearing loss. The size of the tympanic membrane perforation and the volume of the middle ear and mastoid are the primary factors that determine the extent of the hearing loss. The most common causes of a tympanic membrane perforation include acute otitis media, iatrogenic perforation from pressure equalization tube insertion, and trauma. Most acute tympanic membrane perforations heal spontane-ously, with subsequent resolution of the associated conductive hearing loss. A chronic tympanic membrane perforation can be repaired using a variety of techniques; however, a residual conductive hearing loss may persist despite successful closure of the perforation. A tympanic membrane perforation should be readily apparent with a standard otoscopic examination.[49]

CHOLESTEATOMA

A cholesteatoma is the presence of squamous epithelium in the middle ear or mastoid. A congenital cholesteatoma originates from failed involution of middle epithelium during fetal development. Primary acquired cholesteatoma arises from retraction of the tympanic membrane into the middle ear space. Negative middle ear pressure from eustachian tube dysfunction or chronic otitis media is the most common inciting event for tympanic membrane retraction. Secondary acquired cholesteatoma arises when squamous epithelium either migrates into the middle ear from a tympanic membrane perforation or is implanted into the middle ear or mastoid during otologic surgery. Once the skin enters the middle ear or mastoid, normal epithelial migration is interrupted, which results in formation of keratin debris. The accumulated keratin debris are an ideal environment for bacterial proliferation, which results in inflammation and secretion of osteolytic enzymes.[50]

Malodorous otorrhea, progressive hearing loss, tinnitus, otalgia, and rarely dizziness and facial weakness are the typical presenting symptoms in patients with cholesteatoma. Cholesteatoma-mediated hearing loss is most commonly conductive and results from erosion of the ossicular chain. In rare cases, cholesteatoma may erode into the inner ear, resulting in SNHL and dizziness.[51] A thorough otoscopy or binocular microscopy examination is typically all that is necessary to establish the presence of a cholesteatoma. The examiner should pay particular attention to the superior portion of the tympanic membrane, because this is the most common location for cholesteatoma.[52] Obtaining an audiogram is crucial for determining the extent of hearing loss. Temporal bone CT can assist the clinician in determining the extent of cholesteatoma. Removal of the keratin debris and application of combination antibiotic/steroid drops or powders is often all that is necessary to temporarily resolve the malodorous otorrhea. Office debridement of the accumulated keratin may be used in selected cases because most patients require mastoid tympanoplasty surgery to remove the cholesteatoma and to reconstruct the tympanic membrane and ossicular chain. These patients need to be followed carefully with clinical examination and occasionally imaging studies because the cholesteatoma recurrence rates can be as high as 40%.[53]

OTOSCLEROSIS

Otosclerosis, despite being rare, is one of the more common causes of progressive conductive hearing loss in adults who have no prior otologic history (ie, middle ear infections, tympanic membrane perforation, or previous placement of pressure equalization tubes). Otosclerosis is a disorder of bone that is isolated to the inner ear. The mobility of the stapes footplate at its articulation to the vestibule is impaired secondary to osseous fixation to the otic capsule. The impaired mobility of the stapes results in a conductive hearing loss. Extension of the otosclerosis to involve the cochlea results in SNHL in some patients. The onset of otosclerosis typically occurs in the third and fourth decade of life and can rarely present in childhood. Otoscopy reveals a normal-appearing tympanic membrane, but a Weber tuning fork examination typically lateralizes to the most affected ear. Bone conduction is often greater than air conduction on Rinne tuning fork test in patients with more extensive hearing loss.[54]

Several treatment options exist for otosclerosis-related hearing loss, including amplification with a hearing aid, stapedectomy, bone-anchored hearing aids, and rarely cochlear implantation in patients with extensive cochlear involvement with resultant profound SNHL.[55]

TREATMENT

Various options exist of rehabilitation of hearing loss, including hearing aids, assistive listening devices, cochlear implantation, and middle ear surgery. Hearing aids and assistive listening devices function by amplifying ambient sound. Patients with conductive, sensorineural, or mixed hearing loss are candidates for amplification with a hearing aid depending on the configuration and severity of the hearing loss. Hearing aids have been shown in recent studies to improve the social, psychological, emotional, and physical aspects of life in patients with hearing loss. Expense, appearance, and unrealistic expectations are just some of the reasons why only approximately 20% of individuals who would benefit from amplification own a hearing aid. Several factors need to be considered when fitting a hearing aid, including shape of the ear, manual dexterity, cerumen production, condition of the ear, and degree and configuration of hearing loss.[56]

Assistive listening devices can help patients with impaired hearing in various settings. Television devices allow the user to hear directly from the unit using an infrared signal, listening loops for those with hearing aids, or a wired connection with headphones. Devices that assist patients with hearing loss to use the telephone include telecoils for patients with hearing aids and message screens or printouts for patients with profound hearing loss.[57]

A cochlear implant is typically offered to patients with severe to profound SNHL; this is not amenable to amplification with hearing aids. As opposed to hearing aids that amplify sound, cochlear implants function by directly stimulating the eighth cranial nerve. The cochlear implant consists of a surgically implanted internal receiver stimulator and an externally worn speech processor. The speech processor converts sound into its basic frequency components and transmits this information to the internal device, which then directly stimulates the eighth nerve via an electrode implanted into the cochlear lumen.[58]

Middle ear surgery is another means to rehabilitate hearing in selected situations. Tympanic membrane perforations can be repaired, which typically results in improvement or resolution in the associated conductive hearing loss. A stapedectomy for otosclerosis is one of the more successful operations to ameliorate conductive hearing loss. Ossicular chain reconstruction with autologous materials or implants can be successful in improving conductive hearing loss in patients in whom the connection from the tympanic membrane to the stapes footplate has been interrupted.[59]

SUMMARY

Hearing loss is a common and ubiquitous problem that affects individuals of all ages. A significant number of patients presenting to a physician's office report issues related to hearing loss. The differential diagnosis of a patient presenting with hearing loss is vast, but can often be narrowed with an appropriate history and physical examination. Many of these patients benefit from an audiometric assessment and possible intervention depending on the cause and severity of the hearing loss.

REFERENCES

1. Davis AC. Epidemiological profile of hearing impairments: the scale and nature of the problem with special reference to the elderly. Acta Otolaryngol Suppl 1990; 476:23–31.

2. Davis AC, Ostri B, Parving A. Longitudinal study of hearing. Acta Otolaryngol Suppl 1990;476:12–22.
3. Hudspeth AJ. How the ear's works work. Nature 1989;341(6241):397–404.
4. Silverman CA. Audiologic assessment and amplification. Prim Care 1998;25(3): 545–81.
5. Marcincuk MC, Roland PS. Geriatric hearing loss. Understanding the causes and providing appropriate treatment. Geriatrics 2002;57(4):44, 48–50, 55–6 passim.
6. Vikram KB, Naseeruddin K. Combined tuning fork tests in hearing loss: explorative clinical study of the patterns. J Otolaryngol 2004;33(4):227–34.
7. Jackler RK, Shapiro MS, Dillon WP, et al. Gadolinium-DTPA enhanced magnetic resonance imaging in acoustic neuroma diagnosis and management. Otolaryngol Head Neck Surg 1990;102(6):670–7.
8. Valvassori GE, Mafee MF, Dobben GD. Computerized tomography of the temporal bone. Laryngoscope 1982;92(5):562–5.
9. Fransen E, Lemkens W, Van lear L, et al. Age-related hearing impairment (ARHI): environmental risk factors and genetic prospects. Exp Gerontol 2003;38(4):353–9.
10. Dobie RA. Noise-induced permanent threshold shifts in the occupational noise and hearing survey: an explanation for elevated risk estimates. Ear Hear 2007; 28(4):580–91.
11. Nordmann AS, Bohne BA, Harding GW. Histopathological differences between temporary and permanent threshold shift. Hear Res 2000;139(1–2):13–30.
12. Borg E, Counter SA. The middle-ear muscles. Sci Am 1989;261(2):74–80.
13. Serra MR, Biassoni EC, Hinalaf M, et al. Program for the conservation and promotion of hearing among adolescents. Am J Audiol 2007;16(2):S158–64.
14. Conlin AE, Parnes LS. Treatment of sudden sensorineural hearing loss: I. A systematic review. Arch Otolaryngol Head Neck Surg 2007;133(6):573–81.
15. Conlin AE, Parnes LS. Treatment of sudden sensorineural hearing loss: II. A meta-analysis. Arch Otolaryngol Head Neck Surg 2007;133(6):582–6.
16. Merchant SN, Adams JC, Nadol JB Jr. Pathophysiology of Meniere's syndrome: are symptoms caused by endolymphatic hydrops? Otol Neurotol 2005;26(1):74–81.
17. Kotimaki J, Sorri M, Aantaa E, et al. Prevalence of Meniere disease in Finland. Laryngoscope 1999;109(5):748–53.
18. Stahle J, Friberg U, Svedberg A. Long-term progression of Meniere's disease. Am J Otol 1989;10(3):170–3.
19. Grant IL, Welling DB. The treatment of hearing loss in Meniere's disease. Otolaryngol Clin North Am 1997;30(6):1123–44.
20. van Deelen GW, Huizing EH. Use of a diuretic (Dyazide) in the treatment of Meniere's disease. A double-blind cross-over placebo-controlled study. ORL J Otorhinolaryngol Relat Spec 1986;48(5):287–92.
21. Fraysse B, Bebear JP, Dubreuil C, et al. Betahistine dihydrochloride versus flunarizine. A double-blind study on recurrent vertigo with or without cochlear syndrome typical of Meniere's disease. Acta Otolaryngol Suppl 1991;490:1–10.
22. Eisenman DJ, Speers R, Telian SA. Labyrinthectomy versus vestibular neurectomy: long-term physiologic and clinical outcomes. Otol Neurotol 2001;22(4): 539–48.
23. Welling DB, Nagaraja HN. Endolymphatic mastoid shunt: a reevaluation of efficacy. Otolaryngol Head Neck Surg 2000;122(3):340–5.
24. Harner SG, Driscoll CL, Harner GW, et al. Long-term follow-up of transtympanic gentamicin for Meniere's syndrome. Otol Neurotol 2001;22(2):210–4.
25. Lustig LR, Yaegle J, Niparko JK, et al. Cochlear implantation in patients with bilateral Meniere's syndrome. Otol Neurotol 2003;24(3):397–403.

26. Mahaley MS Jr, Mettlin C, Natarajan N, et al. Analysis of patterns of care of brain tumor patients in the United States: a study of the brain tumor section of the AANS and the CNS and the commission on cancer of the ACS. Clin Neurosurg 1990;36: 347–52.
27. Nestor JJ, Korol HW, Nutik SL, et al. The incidence of acoustic neuromas. Arch Otolaryngol Head Neck Surg 1988;114(6):680.
28. Selesnick SH, Jackler RK. Atypical hearing loss in acoustic neuroma patients. Laryngoscope 1993;103(4 Pt 1):437–41.
29. Glasscock ME 3rd, Hart MJ, Vrabec JT. Management of bilateral acoustic neuroma. Otolaryngol Clin North Am 1992;25(2):449–69.
30. Matthies C, Samii M. Management of 1000 vestibular schwannomas (acoustic neuromas): clinical presentation. Neurosurgery 1997;40(1):1–9 [discussion: 9–10].
31. Curtin HD, Hirsch WL Jr. Imaging of acoustic neuromas. Otolaryngol Clin North Am 1992;25(3):553–607.
32. Hajioff D, Raut W, Walsh RM, et al. Conservative management of vestibular schwannomas: third review of a 10-year prospective study. Clin Otolaryngol 2008;33(3):255–9.
33. Flickinger JC, Kondziolka D, Niranjan A, et al. Results of acoustic neuroma radio-surgery: an analysis of 5 years' experience using current methods. J Neurosurg 2001;94(1):1–6.
34. Kondziolka D, Lunsford LD, McLaughlin MR, et al. Long-term outcomes after radiosurgery for acoustic neuromas. N Engl J Med 1998;339(20):1426–33.
35. Slattery WH 3rd. Microsurgery after radiosurgery or radiotherapy for vestibular schwannomas. Otolaryngol Clin North Am 2009;42(4):707–15.
36. Noren G. Long-term complications following gamma knife radiosurgery of vestib-ular schwannomas. Stereotact Funct Neurosurg 1998;70(Suppl 1):65–73.
37. Arts HA, Telian SA, El-Kashlan H, et al. Hearing preservation and facial nerve outcomes in vestibular schwannoma surgery: results using the middle cranial fossa approach. Otol Neurotol 2006;27(2):234–41.
38. Wiet RJ, Teixido M, Liang JG. Complications in acoustic neuroma surgery. Otolar-yngol Clin North Am 1992;25(2):389–412.
39. Tange RA. Ototoxicity. Adverse Drug React Toxicol Rev 1998;17(2–3):75–89.
40. Rizzi MD, Hirose K. Aminoglycoside ototoxicity. Curr Opin Otolaryngol Head Neck Surg 2007;15(5):352–7.
41. Brown ED, Chau JK, Atashband S, et al. A systematic review of neonatal toxoplas-mosis exposure and sensorineural hearing loss. Int J Pediatr Otorhinolaryngol 2009;73(5):707–11.
42. Chau J, Atashband S, Chang E, et al. A systematic review of pediatric sensori-neural hearing loss in congenital syphilis. Int J Pediatr Otorhinolaryngol 2009; 73(6):787–92.
43. Lalwani AK, Castelein CM. Cracking the auditory genetic code: nonsyndromic hereditary hearing impairment. Am J Otol 1999;20(1):115–32.
44. Brodie HA, Thompson TC. Management of complications from 820 temporal bone fractures. Am J Otol 1997;18(2):188–97.
45. Rosenfeld RM, Culpepper L, Dogle KJ, et al. Clinical practice guideline: otitis media with effusion. Otolaryngol Head Neck Surg 2004;130(5 Suppl):S95–118.
46. Rosenfeld RM, Brown L, Cannon CR, et al. Clinical practice guideline: acute otitis externa. Otolaryngol Head Neck Surg 2006;134(4 Suppl):S4–23.
47. Roland PS. Chronic external otitis. Ear Nose Throat J 2001;80(6 Suppl):12–6.
48. Roland PS, Smith TL, Schwartz SR, et al. Clinical practice guideline: cerumen impaction. Otolaryngol Head Neck Surg 2008;139(3 Suppl 2):S1–21.

49. Mehta RP, Rosowski JJ, Voss SE, et al. Determinants of hearing loss in perforations of the tympanic membrane. Otol Neurotol 2006;27(2):136–43.
50. Albino AP, Kimmelman CP, Parisier SC. Cholesteatoma: a molecular and cellular puzzle. Am J Otol 1998;19(1):7–19.
51. Sheehy JL, Brackmann DE. Cholesteatoma surgery: management of the labyrinthine fistula–a report of 97 cases. Laryngoscope 1979;89(1):78–87.
52. Jackler RK. The surgical anatomy of cholesteatoma. Otolaryngol Clin North Am 1989;22(5):883–96.
53. Vartiainen E. Factors associated with recurrence of cholesteatoma. J Laryngol Otol 1995;109(7):590–2.
54. Chole RA, McKenna M. Pathophysiology of otosclerosis. Otol Neurotol 2001; 22(2):249–57.
55. Shea JJ Jr. Forty years of stapes surgery. Am J Otol 1998;19(1):52–5.
56. Larson VD, Williams DW, Henderson WG, et al. A multi-center, double blind clinical trial comparing benefit from three commonly used hearing aid circuits. Ear Hear 2002;23(4):269–76.
57. Lesner SA. Candidacy and management of assistive listening devices: special needs of the elderly. Int J Audiol 2003;42(Suppl 2):2S68–76.
58. Sprinzl GM, Riechelmann H. Current trends in treating hearing loss in elderly people: a review of the technology and treatment options–a mini-review. Gerontology 2010;56(3):351–8.
59. Brenski AC, Isaacson B. Reconstruction of the ossicular chain in children. Operat Tech Otolaryngol Head Neck Surg 2009;20(3):187–96.

The Dizzy Patient

Joe Walter Kutz Jr, MD

KEYWORDS

• Dizziness • Vertigo • Meniere's disease
• Benign positional vertigo • Vestibular neuritis

Functional balance relies on the complex interaction of vestibular function, vision, and proprioception. A defect in any of these areas results in the sensation of imbalance, disequilibrium, light-headedness, or vertigo. The dizzy patient often presents a challenge to the physician. Only through thoughtful history taking, a skillful physical examination, careful selection and interpretation of diagnostic tests, and narrowing down an extensive differential diagnosis can the physician reach a plausible diagnosis.

PHYSIOLOGY

The peripheral vestibular system is composed of 3 semicircular canals and 2 otolith organs, the utricle and saccule. The 3 semicircular canals are arranged in an orthogonal manner and respond to angular head movement. Each canal has a dilated end called the ampulla that consists of vestibular hair cells in the cristae ampullaris and a sail-like structure called the cupula. The hair cells have a single kinocilium and multiple stereocilia that are embedded in the cupula. With head movement, the inertia of the endolymph moves the cupula, which in turn displaces the stereocilia. When the stereocilia are displaced toward the kinocilium, the firing rate of the hair cells increases, and when the stereocilia are displaced away from the kinocilium, the firing rate decreases. Each semicircular canal is paired with the contralateral semicircular canal, resulting in a redundancy to the system that allows for compensation in a unilateral vestibular deficit. The 2 lateral canals are paired, and the superior and contralateral posterior canals are paired (**Fig. 1**). The otolith organs consist of the utricle and saccule and respond to gravitational and translational movement. These organs also have vestibular hair cells with a kinocilium and multiple stereocilia embedded in the otolith membrane. Pathology of the peripheral vestibular system usually results in the sensation of vertigo. Vertigo is different from other sensations of dizziness and is defined as the sensation of movement of the environment or self.

The central vestibular system obtains input from the semicircular canals through the superior and inferior divisions of the vestibular nerve and synapses with the vestibular nuclei. Here, second-order neurons travel ipsilateral and contralateral through the

No funding support.
Department of Otolaryngology, University of Texas Southwestern Medical Center, 5323 Harry Hines Boulevard, Dallas, TX 75390-9035, USA
E-mail address: walter.kutz@utsouthwestern.edu

Med Clin N Am 94 (2010) 989–1002
doi:10.1016/j.mcna.2010.05.011
0025-7125/10/$ – see front matter © 2010 Elsevier Inc. All rights reserved.

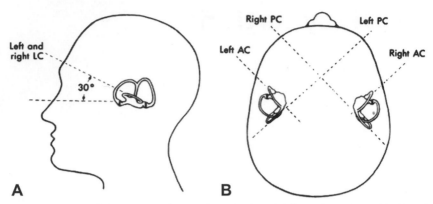

Fig. 1. Orientation of the semicircular canals in the head. (*A*) The lateral canal (LC) is tilted 30° upward from horizontal plane at its anterior end. (*B*) The vertical canals (AC [anterior canal] and PC [posterior canal]) are oriented at roughly 45° from the midsagittal plane. (*From* Barber HO, Stockwell CW. Manual of electronystagmography, St Louis (MO): Mosby-Year Book; 1976. p. 22; with permission.)

medial longitudinal fasciculus to innervate the ocular muscles. This pathway results in the vestibuloocular reflex (VOR), which is responsible for maintaining vision on an object during fast head movements. The utricle and saccule send information through the superior and inferior vestibular nerves to the vestibular nuclei as well. However, the second-order neurons of the otolith organs primarily send information to the cervical, spinal, and lower extremity muscles to adjust to changes in translational or gravitational forces. The cerebellum is responsible for fine tuning motor activity and coordinating vestibular, visual, and somatosensory input. Rapid changes in eye position in response to changes in the visual field are referred to as saccades and are generated in the frontal lobe. Smooth pursuit is used to track slow objects in space and relies on the input from the visual cortex to the vestibular nucleus. Smooth pursuit declines with age, sedation, inattention, and changes in visual acuity.

HISTORY

A thorough and thoughtful history is the most important component during the evaluation of the dizzy patient (**Table 1**). The first goal is to determine if the patient is experiencing vertigo, the sensation of movement, or some other sensation, such as lightheadedness, imbalance, disequilibrium, or near-syncope. Once this is determined, the cause of the dizziness can often be categorized as peripheral or central. The second question to address is the nature of the dizziness and whether it is episodic or persistent. If the dizziness is episodic, the length of the episodes should be determined. Peripheral causes of dizziness rarely last more than a day. If the dizziness is persistent or lasts for more than a day, a central vestibular disorder is likely. Patients are asked if they can recall the first episode and to recall the inciting factors, duration, and severity of the episode. In peripheral vestibular disorders, the dizziness is severe enough for the patients to recall the first episode, whereas central vestibular disorders more often present with an insidious onset.

Associated symptoms should be identified and can often narrow the differential diagnosis. Peripheral vestibular disorders are often associated with hearing loss, tinnitus, aural fullness, and nausea. For instance, fluctuating hearing loss, tinnitus,

Table 1
Clinical features distinguishing peripheral and central causes of dizziness

Clinical Feature	Peripheral	Central
Onset	Sudden	Gradual
Duration of episodes	Seconds to hours, rarely greater than 24 h	Seconds to days
Visceral symptoms (nausea, vomiting, diaphoresis)	Yes	Rarely
Auditory symptoms (hearing loss, tinnitus, aural fullness)	Often	Rarely
Neurologic symptoms	Rarely	Often
Nystagmus		
Direction	Horizontal and torsional, never vertical	Horizontal, torsional, vertical, and direction changing
Fatigable	Yes	No
Onset	Delayed	Immediate
Decreases with visual fixation	Yes	No

and fullness associated with episodic vertigo is consistent with Meniere's disease. Symptoms of changes in vision, dysarthria, and headaches are associated with central causes of dizziness. Syncope, shortness of breath, and palpitations are most consistent with a cardiovascular cause. Diaphoresis, dyspnea, and feeling of impending doom suggest anxiety disorder or panic attacks.

Past medical and surgical history is an important component of the evaluation of the dizzy patient. A wide variety of comorbid conditions may cause the sensation of dizziness. Cardiovascular disease may cause dizziness because of structural heart disease or abnormalities of the peripheral vascular system. Arrhythmias, coronary artery disease, heart failure, cardiomyopathy, and myocardial infarction may all present with dizziness. Peripheral vascular disease can be divided into problems with vasomotor tone or arterial occlusion. Orthostatic hypotension is common and presents with faintness when the patient stands from a sitting or supine position. This condition can be easily investigated in the office by comparing the blood pressure while lying supine with that while standing. A decrease of greater than 20 mm Hg in systolic pressure after standing for 2 minutes is suggestive of orthostatic hypotension. Atherosclerosis may decrease cerebral blood flow to cause the sensation of faintness.

Diseases affecting the visual system may also result in imbalance and disequilibrium. Patients should be asked about their visual acuity and if they have recently changed the prescription of their glasses. Bifocals and trifocals are often responsible for causing chronic disequilibrium. Binocular image conflict occurs when the image size is different between the two retinas and may cause problems with disequilibrium.

Neurologic disorders such as multiple sclerosis, cerebrovascular disorders, migraines, seizure disorders, meningitis, and peripheral neuropathies may all manifest as dizziness. Approximately 5% of patients with multiple sclerosis present with the initial complaint of dizziness, and up to 50% of patients complain of dizziness during the course of the disease.[1] Cerebrovascular disease affecting the posterior circulation may manifest as dizziness, which can be caused by cerebellar infarction or hemorrhage, cerebellar artery occlusion, or vertebrobasilar insufficiency (VBI).

Aging produces many degenerative changes that affect balance. The peripheral vestibular system is affected by the degeneration of the ampullae of the semicircular canals and the otolith organs.[2] The vestibular nuclei and brainstem pathways also show a decrease in function with time.[3] Visual acuity usually declines with age, resulting in problems with balance. Proprioception ability decreases because of slower nerve conduction velocities, less-defined 2-point discrimination, and decreased vibratory sensation.[4–6] Many older patients have significant joint disease that results in decreased proprioceptive input.

Medications should be reviewed because antihypertensives, quinolones, neuroleptics, antidepressants, sedatives, and anticonvulsants can cause central vestibular dysfunction. In addition, polypharmacy is a common cause of dizziness, especially in elderly patients and may need a geriatrician to coordinate the patient's care to decrease the amount of needed medication. Medications that may cause dizziness because of effects on the peripheral vestibular system include aminoglycosides, alkylating agents and cyclophosphamide, aspirin, nonsteroidal antiinflammatory drugs, loop diuretics, and quinines. Aminoglycoside antibiotics may destroy the auditory and vestibular hair cells and are the most common cause for drug-induced bilateral vestibulopathy. Vestibulotoxicity depends on drug concentration, length of treatment, and renal clearance.[7,8] However, staying within therapeutic levels does not ensure prevention of vestibulotoxicity.[9] If a patient is taking an aminoglycoside antibiotic and begins to show signs of hearing loss or imbalance, the antibiotic should be stopped immediately because the damage to hair cells can be permanent.[10]

PHYSICAL EXAMINATION

All components of the balance system should be examined, including the peripheral vestibular system, central vestibular system, visual system, proprioception, and the interactions between these systems. It is important to perform a thorough physical examination to detect uncommon or multiple causes of dizziness.

The physical examination begins with a general assessment of the patient. It should be noticed if the patient is ambulating using an assistive device, such as a cane or walker. The use of glasses may suggest an ocular cause of dizziness. Facial asymmetry, dysarthria, and hoarseness may suggest a cerebrovascular accident or tumor as the cause of dizziness. Vital signs should be obtained, including blood pressure, in the supine and sitting positions to evaluate for orthostatic hypotension. The peripheral pulse should be examined to evaluate for tachycardia or arrhythmias.

An otoscopic examination is important. Abnormalities possibly encountered include middle ear effusions, tympanic membrane perforations, cholesteatoma, and neoplasms. Pneumatic otoscopy may cause vertigo and nystagmus in patients with perilabyrinthine fistula, Meniere's disease, or superior canal dehiscence. Tuning fork examination, including the Weber and Rinne examination, are essential to evaluate the patient for any hearing loss and to determine if the hearing loss is sensorineural or conductive in nature.

The visual system is examined to evaluate extraocular movements, visual acuity, visual fields, and the fundus. The patient's glasses should be inspected for bifocal or trifocal lenses.

The neurologic examination can be extensive and is often tailored to the differential diagnosis. Nystagmus is an abnormal eye response to vestibular dysfunction through the VOR. For example, if there is a lesion that decreases the neural activity of a horizontal semicircular canal (ie, vestibular neuritis), the VOR causes the eyes to deviate towards from the affected side. In response to that movement, the central vestibular system responds by bringing the eyes back to midline with a fast saccade. By convention, the direction of the nystagmus is determined by the fast phase. Nystagmus can be horizontal, vertical, torsional, or a combination of these directions. Most peripheral vestibulopathies present with horizontal and torsional nystagmus. Vertical nystagmus is almost always associated with a central vestibular disorder. One of the hallmark features of a peripheral vestibular disorder that is not present with central vestibular disorder is the ability to suppress the nystagmus with visual fixation. For this reason, Frenzel glasses consisting of high-diopter lenses are used to evaluate for nystagmus to prevent visual fixation and increase the sensitivity of the examination for nystagmus. This is also the reason that vestibular testing, such as the electronystagmogram (ENG) and rotary chair examinations, are performed in a dark environment.

VOR TESTING

The head thrust test is an easily performed bedside examination that accurately evaluates the VOR.[11,12] History of neck pain or trauma should be elicited and may prevent the physician from performing this test. The patient is asked to keep the eyes focused on the examiner's nose. Quick and unpredictable thrusts of the head to the right and left should be performed, and the eyes should be evaluated for saccades. If the patient has an intact VOR, the eyes remain focused on the examiner's nose. If the examination result is abnormal, a corrective saccade is seen. If the patient has a unilateral peripheral weakness, the corrective saccade occurs with the head turned to the affected side (**Fig. 2**).

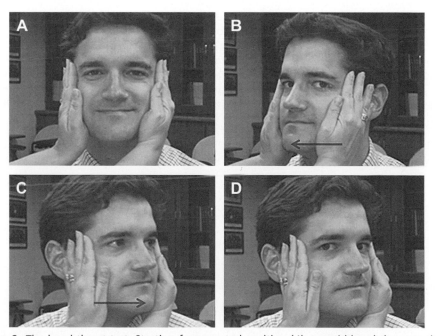

Fig. 2. The head thrust test. Starting from neutral position (*A*), a rapid head thrust to the right in the horizontal plane elicits compensatory eye movements to the left. As a result, the eyes remain fixed on the examiner (*B*). A similar movement to the left with a hypoactive labyrinth (*C*) results in a delayed catchup-saccade (*D*) to maintain gaze on the examiner. (*Courtesy of* Joe Kutz, MD.)

The VOR can also be evaluated by measuring dynamic visual acuity.[13,14] The patient is asked to read a Snellen chart to determine the visual acuity with the head still. They are then asked to rotate their head about 60° in both directions at a frequency of 1 to 2 Hz. Patients with normal vestibular function will have a decrease in visual acuity of about 1 line. Patients with unilateral weakness may experience a decrease in visual acuity of 3 to 4 lines. Patients with bilateral vestibular weakness will have a decrease in visual acuity of 5 to 6 lines. This test is especially valuable as a bedside examination to monitor for aminoglycoside toxicity.

Post–head shaking nystagmus can be used to evaluate the VOR.[15–17] The patient actively or passively shakes the head at a high velocity for 10 to 20 seconds. This activity increases the velocity storage of the central vestibular pathways. When the head shaking stops, the normal patient or a patient with bilateral vestibulopathy should not have significant nystagmus because the velocity storage is symmetric. With a unilateral weakness, the patient demonstrates nystagmus that is initially away from the affected side with a possible reversal phase. In an acute unilateral vestibulopathy, the central vestibular velocity storage system may be clamped down and nystagmus is not present after head shaking.

POSITIONAL TESTING

Positional testing is usually performed using the Dix-Hallpike examination (**Fig. 3**). The patient is seated on an examination table, and the head is turned 30°. The examiner quickly places the patient in the supine position with the head still turned 30° and hanging off the table at a 30° angle. In classic benign paroxysmal positional vertigo (BPPV), nystagmus starts after a latent period of 3 to 5 seconds and lasts for 15 to 20 seconds. The nystagmus is geotropic rotary toward the ground, and the downward ear is the affected ear. Central causes can also cause positional nystagmus of central type. Central causes of positional nystagmus can be differentiated from BPPV because there is usually no latency between the maneuver and the nystagmus, the nystagmus does not fatigue with repeated maneuvers, visual fixation does not decrease the nystagmus, and the nystagmus lasts much longer than seen in BPPV.

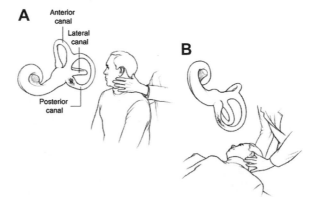

Fig. 3. The Dix-Hallpike maneuver. Lowering the patient's head backward and to the side allows debris in the posterior canal (*A*) to fall to its lowest position, activating the canal and causing eye movements and vertigo (*B*). (*From* Hullar TE, Minor LB. Vestibular physiology and disorders of the labyrinth. In: Glasscock E 3rd, Gulya AJ, editors. Surgery of the ear. 5th edition. Hamilton (Canada): BC Decker; 2003. p. 97; with permission.)

CEREBELLAR FUNCTION

Coordination, gait, and posture should be evaluated. Dysmetria (inability to measure speed, distance, and power of a movement) is determined by asking patients to touch their nose and then touch the tip of the examiner's finger. Dysdiadochokinesis (inability to rapidly change to an opposite movement) is examined by asking the patient to rapidly alternate hand movements. The Romberg examination is useful for testing proprioception and vestibular function. Patients are asked to stand with their feet together and arms either at the side or crossed. Then they are asked to close their eyes and are examined for at least 10 seconds. Patients with a unilateral vestibular weakness tend to fall to the affected side. The sharpened or tandem Romberg examination is more sensitive and similar to the Romberg examination, but the patient is made to place one foot in front of the other. The Fukuda stepping test evaluates for a unilateral vestibular weakness.[16] The patient marches in place with arms extended and eyes closed for at least 50 steps. Normal patients show drift to the left or right of less than 30°; however, patients with a unilateral vestibular weakness drift to the affected side. Finally, the patients' gait should be examined.

VESTIBULAR TESTING

Often the diagnosis of the dizzy patient can be achieved through a thorough history and careful physical examination. However, in select circumstances, vestibular testing may be required to differentiate peripheral from central causes of dizziness, for preoperative evaluation, to determine recovery after a unilateral injury, or to monitor the results of vestibular rehabilitation.

The ENG is the most commonly performed vestibular battery in the evaluation of a dizzy patient. Eye movement is recorded either with surface electrodes or by infrared goggles. The ENG is divided into subtests that measure smooth pursuit, saccades, spontaneous nystagmus, gaze fixation, optokinetic stimulation, positional nystagmus, Dix-Hallpike maneuver, and caloric response. Perhaps the most useful portion of the examination is the caloric test, which can compare caloric responses between sides and is useful for detecting a unilateral vestibular weakness.

The rotary chair testing is done in a darkened enclosure, with the patient sitting on a chair that can be rotated in either direction. Eye movements are recorded in response to movements at different velocities. Rotary chair testing is useful for confirming a bilateral vestibulopathy in patients with bilateral caloric weakness.[18,19] It is also useful to determine incomplete compensation after a vestibular injury.[20]

BLOOD TESTS

Routine blood tests are not cost-effective.[21] However, selective blood tests may be obtained with a supporting history. Complete blood count, levels of electrolytes, cholesterol panel, and thyroid function studies may be considered in patients with an unclear cause for dizziness. In patients with vertigo and fluctuating bilateral hearing loss, an autoimmune panel and tests for syphilis should be obtained.

IMAGING OF THE DIZZY PATIENT

Patients with a typical history of peripheral causes of vertigo, such as BPPV or vestibular neuritis, do not normally need imaging. Patients with asymmetric hearing loss, with central causes of dizziness with unclear causes, and presenting with other neurologic signs should undergo imaging.

Magnetic resonance imaging (MRI) with gadolinium contrast is the most common imaging modality used to evaluate the dizzy patient. Cerebellopontine lesions, such as vestibular schwannomas and meningiomas, are easily diagnosed with gadolinium-enhanced MRI. Multiple sclerosis can present with hyperintense plaques seen on fluid-attenuated inversion recovery and T2-weighted images. Acute or chronic ischemic disease is easily diagnosed with MRI.

Computed tomography (CT) complements the MRI because of the superior imaging of the bony labyrinth. If a semicircular canal fistula is suspected as the cause of dizziness (patient has vertigo with loud noise or with Valsalva maneuver), CT can confirm this diagnosis. Superior semicircular canal dehiscence was first described in 1998 by Minor and colleagues[22] and causes pressure- and/or sound-induced vertigo. This diagnosis is confirmed with high-resolution CT (**Fig. 4**). Temporal bone fractures are best evaluated with CT and can show a fracture extending across the otic capsule and involving the labyrinth.

SPECIFIC DISORDERS CAUSING DIZZINESS
Peripheral Causes of Vertigo

BPPV
BPPV is the most common cause of vertigo and is caused by the dislodgement of otoconia from the utricle. The otoconial debris usually migrates into the posterior semicircular canal, although the lateral semicircular canal may be affected in about 10% of cases. The patient experiences intense vertigo with head movement toward the affected ear and when looking upward. The vertigo is characterized by a latency of a few seconds from the movement until the onset of vertigo, vertigo lasting less than 1 minute, decreased intensity of vertigo with successive inciting head movement (fatigue), and visual suppression. The Dix-Hallpike examination is used to test for BPPV. Patients are asked to turn their heads about 30° to 45° to the side while sitting. The examiner quickly lays the patient supine with the head kept at the 45° and extended about 30° below the level of the examination table. The nystagmus is torsional and occurs when the head is turned toward the affected side. Repositioning maneuvers, such as the Epley maneuver, significantly improve symptoms in

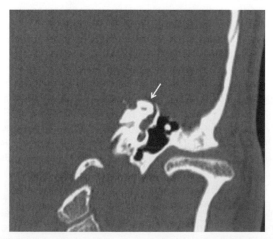

Fig. 4. High-resolution CT parallel to the plane of the superior semicircular canal. The arrow points to the area of dehiscence.

approximately 90% of patients.[23,24] Without treatment, symptoms usually resolve within 6 months, although the condition can be recurrent. In recurrent or persistent cases, despite repositioning exercises, surgical plugging of the posterior semicircular canal may be performed.[25]

Meniere's disease

Meniere's disease is characterized by fluctuating low-frequency hearing loss, episodic vertigo, aural fullness, and tinnitus. The vertigo episodes typically last for hours and rarely last for more than a day. The episodes are severe and are often accompanied by nausea, vomiting, and diaphoresis. Spontaneous remission and exacerbations are typical. Meniere's disease usually affects 1 ear but may be bilateral in 17% of patients.[26]

The cause and pathophysiology of Meniere's disease is poorly understood. The common histologic finding is evidence of elevated endolymph pressure that may be because of excessive endolymph production, decreased endolymph resorption, altered glycoprotein metabolism, or immune-mediated inner ear disease.[27] These conditions may be caused by viral infection, allergies, genetic factors, or trauma. The increased endolymph pressure causes breaks in the intralabyrinthine membranes, resulting in vertigo. The increased pressure also results in the fluctuating hearing loss that can progress to severe hearing loss In the affected ear.

Dietary changes consisting of a low-salt diet (<1500 mg daily) and low-caffeine diet is the most common first-line treatment and results in adequate treatment for most patients.[28,29] Medical therapy consisting of a diuretic and benzodiazepines to treat acute episodes along with the aforementioned dietary changes controls symptoms in approximately 80% of patients. For the 20% of patients who fail dietary and medical therapy, multiple surgical and nonsurgical interventions exist. Nonablative treatment options include intratympanic steroid injection, surgical decompression of the endo-lymphatic sac, or the use of a daily low-pressure pulse generator (Meniett Device, Medtronic USA, Inc, Jacksonville, FL, USA). Ablative therapies include intratympanic gentamicin injection (chemical labyrinthectomy), labyrinthectomy, or vestibular nerve section. More than 95% of patients experience a significant reduction of vertigo with stepwise treatment consisting of these options. Hearing loss and tinnitus are more difficult to treat.

Vestibular neuritis and labyrinthitis

Vestibular neuritis is characterized by intense vertigo lasting for a few days followed by disequilibrium and imbalance lasting for days to weeks. If hearing loss is also present, a diagnosis of labyrinthitis is made. The diagnosis is made by the characteristic history and by excluding other causes of dizziness. ENG shows a decreased response of the affected labyrinth through caloric stimulation. MRI may demonstrate enhancement of the eighth cranial nerve or labyrinth. The condition is thought to occur either because of a viral infection causing inflammation or because of vascular occlusion.[30–32]

Vestibular suppressants such as meclizine and benzodiazepines may be used during the acute phase of vertigo; however, the use of vestibular suppressants for more than a week should be avoided to prevent poor compensation. There is evidence that oral steroids may show benefit, if used during the acute phase.[33] Most patients recover over the ensuing weeks, and vestibular rehabilitation is an important treatment for patients who show slow or poor recovery. Patients with vestibular neuritis are at a higher risk of developing BPPV. Treatment with canalith repositioning maneuvers is usually successful in resolving the positional vertigo.

Vestibular schwannoma (acoustic neuroma)

Cerebellopontine angle masses, such as vestibular schwannomas and meningiomas, may present with dizziness and, less commonly, vertigo. Vestibular schwannomas and meningiomas are easily detected by gadolinium-enhanced MRI. Treatment varies from observation, radiosurgery, or surgical resection with or without hearing preservation.

Superior canal dehiscence syndrome

Superior canal dehiscence syndrome was first described in 1998 by Minor and colleagues.[22] Patients present with sound- and/or pressure-induced vertigo. Other complaints include hearing bodily sounds, such as eye or neck motion; a conductive hearing loss; and autophony (hearing one's voice). Dehiscence of the superior semicircular canal is diagnosed by high-resolution CT in planes perpendicular and parallel to the superior semicircular canal. Patients significantly affected by the symptoms may undergo plugging of the superior semicircular canal.

Trauma

Trauma may result in multiple causes for dizziness, such as BPPV, labyrinthine concussion, temporal bone fractures involving the otic capsule, perilymph fistula (PLF), or endolymphatic hydrops (increased pressure of the endolymph).

PLF is a communication of the perilymph to the middle ear. Patients often have a sensorineural hearing loss that may fluctuate and a constant disequilibrium. Usually the disequilibrium subsides with bed rest and conservative measures, although the hearing loss may be permanent. A middle ear exploration and grafting of the oval and round windows may be performed if the patient develops persistent disequilibrium despite conservative measures.

Labyrinthine concussion is characterized by the immediate onset of vertigo after trauma. The vertigo usually lasts for several days and is followed by a period of dizziness lasting for several weeks. If symptoms do not resolve over several weeks, avoidance of vestibular suppressants and vestibular rehabilitation may be beneficial. Delayed endolymphatic hydrops may occur years after trauma and presents with the same symptoms as Meniere's disease.

Ototoxicity

Ototoxicity may occur with the use of topical or systemic therapies. Otic drops containing polymyxin B and neomycin are ototoxic and should be avoided in patients without an intact tympanic membrane. Topical aminoglycosides are ototoxic, affecting hearing and balance. If there is a question of a tympanic membrane perforation or a tympanostomy tube in place, a fluoroquinolone antibiotic drop should be used.

Systemic aminoglycoside therapy may result in ototoxicity affecting the auditory and vestibular systems. The changes are subtle, and the patient may not notice hearing loss or imbalance until significant changes occur. If the vestibular system is affected, both labyrinths will be affected, resulting in a bilateral vestibular weakness. Patients complain of oscillopsia (objects appear to oscillate) and have difficulty walking in the dark. The most useful method for preventing ototoxicity from aminoglycoside antibiotics is the use of an alternative antibiotic if possible or careful monitoring for ototoxicity through audiograms or vestibular testing. Confirming serum levels of the aminoglycoside to be within therapeutic range does not necessarily prevent ototoxicity.

Central Causes of Dizziness

Migraine-associated dizziness

Vertigo is a common symptom in patients with migraines. Kayan and Hood[34] reported that 27% of patients with migraines suffered vertigo compared with an incidence of 8% in patients with tension headaches. In addition, the vertigo episodes are often separate from the headaches.[35,36] Unlike Meniere's disease, the vertigo episodes may last for more than a day at a time. Other characteristic features include a family history of migraines, motion intolerance, and sensitivity to visual stimuli.[36]

Treatment involves dietary modifications and migraine prophylaxis medications, including tricyclic antidepressants, topiramate, calcium-channel blockers, and β-blockers.[37] Abortive medications, such as the triptans, are usually not effective in treating the vertigo episodes.

Vascular insufficiency syndromes

Vertebrobasilar insufficiency (VBI) results in transient ischemia of the posterior cerebral circulation, resulting in vertigo usually lasting minutes. Additional neurologic signs, including dysarthria, numbness of the face, hemiparesis, headache, diplopia, visual field defects, blindness, dysphagia, ataxia, and drops attacks, may also be present. If compression occurs secondary to cervical spondylosis, vertigo may be triggered with a head turn. Treatment of this condition consists of antiplatelet therapy or aggressive anticoagulation in patients with progressive symptoms.

Multiple sclerosis

Approximately 5% to 7% of patients with multiple sclerosis present with acute vertigo.[38,39] However, balance disturbances may occur in up to 78% of patients with multiple sclerosis.[40] Multiple areas along the vestibular pathways may be affected, including the eighth nerve, vestibular nuclei, oculomotor tracts, medial longitudinal fasciculus, and the cerebellum. MRI evaluation often shows characteristic demyelinating plaques.

Cervical vertigo and trauma

Trauma may result in a postconcussion syndrome that is characterized by a constant disequilibrium. If the cervical muscles are involved, such as in a whiplash injury, the patient may complain of constant disequilibrium and restricted neck movement. Often a trigger point can be found in the cervical muscles that replicates the symptoms. Treatment for cervical vertigo is physical therapy.

Mal de debarquement syndrome

Mal de debarquement typically occurs after a long sea voyage, such as a cruise. However, it may also begin after any long trip by car, plane, or train. The condition is characterized by a constant feeling of swaying, as if one were still on the boat. The condition is most common in women in their 40s. The symptoms can last from months to years, with an average length of symptoms of 3.5 years.[41] Some patients benefit from low-dose benzodiazepine therapy.

Orthostatic hypotension

Orthostatic hypotension should be considered in patients who develop feelings of dizziness, light-headedness, or near syncope with changes in position. An easy bedside examination is performed by comparing the blood pressure while lying supine with that while standing for 2 minutes. Patients with orthostatic hypotension usually experience dizziness and a decrease in the systolic blood pressure by greater than

20 mm Hg. Common causes for orthostatic hypotension include diabetic autonomic neuropathy and antihypertensive medications.

Psychogenic dizziness

Many patients who present with dizziness do not fall within a typical diagnosis. Staab and Ruckenstein[42] found that 60% of patients who were referred for chronic dizziness of uncertain cause had either a primary or a secondary anxiety disorder. Patients with anxiety disorder often demonstrate symptoms in open places, such as concert halls or large stores. Symptoms can be replicated by making the patient to hyperventilate.

SUMMARY

The dizzy patient often presents a challenge to the physician. A careful understanding of the history is the most important component of the evaluation and should result in categorizing the dizziness as peripheral or central. Peripheral dizziness is characterized by a sensation of movement (vertigo). The vertigo is usually paroxysmal and episodic, associated with visceral symptoms such as nausea, and sometimes associated with hearing loss, aural fullness, or tinnitus. Central dizziness is more often constant, insidious, and less severe.

A plausible diagnosis to explain the patient's dizziness can often be reached with a thorough history taking and physical examination. However, if a clear diagnosis is not made, further investigation with vestibular testing, imaging, and laboratory evaluation may be needed. MRI is the most important imaging modality to evaluate for tumors, cerebrovascular causes, and other central causes, such as multiple sclerosis. Vestibular testing may be required to differentiate peripheral causes from central causes of dizziness, for preoperative evaluation, to determine recovery after a unilateral injury, or to monitor the results of vestibular rehabilitation.

Topical or systemic ototoxic medications are a common cause of vestibular dysfunction and should be avoided or closely monitored. Topical antibiotics containing polymyxin B, neomycin, or an aminoglycoside should not be used in patients with a tympanic membrane perforation or a tympanostomy tube. Avoidance of aminoglycoside ototoxicity is not necessarily preventable by keeping serum levels at therapeutic levels. An alternative antibiotic is the best prevention for ototoxicity.

In most cases, vestibular suppressant medications, such as scopolamine, meclizine, and benzodiazepines, should be avoided. Prolonged use results in delayed or poor central compensation. Vestibular rehabilitation is helpful for most conditions characterized by chronic imbalance.

REFERENCES

1. Grénman R. Involvement of the audiovestibular system in multiple sclerosis. An otoneurologic and audiologic study. Acta Otolaryngol Suppl 1985;420:1–95.
2. Rauch SD, Velazquez-Villaseñor L, Dimitri PS, et al. Decreasing hair cell counts in aging humans. Ann N Y Acad Sci 2001;942:220–7.
3. Hirvonen TP, Aalto H, Pyykkö I, et al. Changes in vestibulo-ocular reflex of elderly people. Acta Otolaryngol Suppl 1997;529:108–10.
4. Kaneko A, Asai N, Kanda T. The influence of age on pressure perception of static and moving two-point discrimination in normal subjects. J Hand Ther 2005;18(4): 421–4 [quiz: 425].
5. Shimokata H, Kuzuya F. Two-point discrimination test of the skin as an index of sensory aging. Gerontology 1995;41(5):267–72.

6. Taylor PK. Non-linear effects of age on nerve conduction in adults. J Neurol Sci 1984;66(2–3):223–34.
7. Black FO, Pesznecker S, Stallings V. Permanent gentamicin vestibulotoxicity. Otol Neurotol 2004;25(4):559–69.
8. Schwartz FD. Vestibular toxicity of gentamicin in the presence of renal disease. Arch Intern Med 1978;138(11):1612–3.
9. Halmagyi GM, Fattore CM, Curthoys IS, et al. Gentamicin vestibulotoxicity. Otolaryngol Head Neck Surg 1994;111(5):571–4.
10. Black FO, Gianna-Poulin C, Pesznecker SC. Recovery from vestibular ototoxicity. Otol Neurotol 2001;22(5):662–71.
11. Weber KP, Aw ST, Todd MJ, et al. Head impulse test in unilateral vestibular loss: vestibulo-ocular reflex and catch-up saccades. Neurology 2008;70(6):454–63.
12. Roy FD, Tomlinson RD. Characterization of the vestibulo-ocular reflex evoked by high-velocity movements. Laryngoscope 2004;114(7):1190–3.
13. Dannenbaum E, Paquet N, Chilingaryan G, et al. Clinical evaluation of dynamic visual acuity in subjects with unilateral vestibular hypofunction. Otol Neurotol 2009;30(3):368–72.
14. Demer JL, Honrubia V, Baloh RW. Dynamic visual acuity: a test for oscillopsia and vestibulo-ocular reflex function. Am J Otol 1994;15(3):340–7.
15. Tseng HZ, Chao WY. Head-shaking nystagmus: a sensitive indicator of vestibular dysfunction. Clin Otolaryngol Allied Sci 1997;22(6):549–52.
16. Fukuda T. The stepping test: two phases of the labyrinthine reflex. Acta Otolaryngol 1959;50(2):95–108.
17. Vicini C, Casani A, Ghilardi P. Assessment of head shaking test in neuro-otological practice. ORL J Otorhinolaryngol Relat Spec 1989;51(1):8–13.
18. Telian SA, Shepard NT, Smith-Wheelock M, et al. Bilateral vestibular paresis: diagnosis and treatment. Otolaryngol Head Neck Surg 1991;104(1):67–71.
19. Furman JM, Kamerer DB. Rotational responses in patients with bilateral caloric reduction. Acta Otolaryngol 1989;108(5–6):355–61.
20. Myers SF. Patterns of low-frequency rotational responses in bilateral caloric weakness patients. J Vestib Res 1992;2(2):123–31.
21. Stewart MG, Chen AY, Wyatt JR, et al. Cost-effectiveness of the diagnostic evaluation of vertigo. Laryngoscope 1999;109(4):600–5.
22. Minor LB, Solomon D, Zinreich JS, et al. Sound- and/or pressure-induced vertigo due to bone dehiscence of the superior semicircular canal. Arch Otolaryngol Head Neck Surg 1998;124(3):249–58.
23. Richard W, Bruintjes TD, Oostenbrink P, et al. Efficacy of the Epley maneuver for posterior canal BPPV: a long-term, controlled study of 81 patients. Ear Nose Throat J 2005;84(1):22–5.
24. Epley JM. The canalith repositioning procedure: for treatment of benign paroxysmal positional vertigo. Otolaryngol Head Neck Surg 1992;107(3):399–404.
25. Parnes LS, McClure JA. Posterior semicircular canal occlusion for intractable benign paroxysmal positional vertigo. Ann Otol Rhinol Laryngol 1990;99(5 Pt 1):330–4.
26. House JW, Doherty JK, Fisher LM, et al. Meniere's disease: prevalence of contralateral ear involvement. Otol Neurotol 2006;27(3):355–61.
27. Wackym PA, Sando I. Molecular and cellular pathology of Meniere's disease. Otolaryngol Clin North Am 1997;30(6):947–60.
28. van Deelen GW, Huizing EH. Use of a diuretic (Dyazide) in the treatment of Menière's disease. A double-blind cross-over placebo-controlled study. ORL J Otorhinolaryngol Relat Spec 1986;48(5):287–92.

29. Klockhoff I, Lindblom U. Menière's disease and hydrochlorothiazide (Dichlotride)—a critical analysis of symptoms and therapeutic effects. Acta Otolaryngol 1967;63(4):347–65.
30. Arbusow V, Schulz P, Strupp M, et al. Distribution of herpes simplex virus type 1 in human geniculate and vestibular ganglia: implications for vestibular neuritis. Ann Neurol 1999;46(3):416–9.
31. Furuta Y, Takasu T, Fukuda S, et al. Latent herpes simplex virus type 1 in human vestibular ganglia. Acta Otolaryngol Suppl 1993;503:85–9.
32. Friedmann I, House W. Vestibular neuronitis. Electron microscopy of Scarpa's ganglion. J Laryngol Otol 1980;94(8):877–83.
33. Kitahara T, Kondoh K, Morihana T, et al. Steroid effects on vestibular compensation in human. Neurol Res 2003;25(3):287–91.
34. Kayan A, Hood JD. Neuro-otological manifestations of migraine. Brain 1984; 107(Pt 4):1123–42.
35. Cutrer FM, Baloh RW. Migraine-associated dizziness. Headache 1992;32(6): 300–4.
36. Kuritzky A, Ziegler DK, Hassanein R. Vertigo, motion sickness and migraine. Headache 1981;21(5):227–31.
37. Reploeg MD, Goebel JA. Migraine-associated dizziness: patient characteristics and management options. Otol Neurotol 2002;23:364–71.
38. Herrera WG. Vestibular and other balance disorders in multiple sclerosis. Differential diagnosis of disequilibrium and topognostic localization. Neurol Clin 1990; 8(2):407–20.
39. Kahana E, Leibowitz U, Alter M. Brainstem and cranial nerve involvement in multiple sclerosis. Acta Neurol Scand 1973;49(3):269–79.
40. Muller R. Studies on disseminated sclerosis with special reference to symptomatology, course and prognosis. Acta Med Scand 1949;133(Suppl 222):1–214.
41. Hain TC, Hanna PA, Rheinberger MA. Mal de debarquement. Arch Otolaryngol Head Neck Surg 1999;125(6):615–20.
42. Staab JP, Ruckenstein MJ. Expanding the differential diagnosis of chronic dizziness. Arch Otolaryngol Head Neck Surg 2007;133(2):170–6.

The Patient with a Thyroid Nodule

Matthew C. Miller, MD

KEYWORDS

• Thyroid nodule • Fine-needle aspiration • Incidentaloma
• Thyroidectomy

As defined by the American Thyroid Association's task force on the management of thyroid nodules and differentiated thyroid cancer,[1] a thyroid nodule is "a discrete lesion within the thyroid gland that is radiologically distinct from the surrounding thyroid parenchyma." By this definition, nodular thyroid disease is common in the United States and throughout the world. With increased sensitivities of radiographic studies, it is expected that the prevalence of thyroid nodules will also rise.

Although most nodules are benign and asymptomatic, there is a small but not insignificant risk of carcinoma that necessitates further evaluation in many patients – including the consideration for surgical intervention. This article familiarizes the reader with a number of the current concepts pertaining to nodular thyroid disease and provides a framework for appropriate diagnostic evaluation and referral to an endocrine or head and neck surgeon.

RISK FACTORS FOR THE DEVELOPMENT OF THYROID NODULES

Several authors have attempted to establish risk factors for the development of solitary nodules and nonendemic multinodular disease. The most comprehensive and systematic evaluation of these was published by Knudsen and colleagues[2] in 2002. Their cohort of 4649 Danish patients was evaluated in the context of other large series and a set of risk factors for both goiter and thyroid nodules was proposed. In Knudsen's and other similar papers, the strongest of these were female gender, tobacco smoking, and advanced age.[2–4] Interestingly, subset analysis found that most of the age-related prevalence differences were attributable to the presence of multinodular disease.[2] Other individual studies have pointed to radiation exposure as a risk factor for nodules. Although radiation-induced thyroid disease is generally thought to be associated with childhood exposure,[5] relative risk rates may also be as high as eight times in occupationally exposed adults.[6] As indicated by the gender disparity in thyroid nodule risk, hormonal influences may also be at play. Pregnancy and multiparity are associated with an increase in the size of pre-existing nodules and with the

Department of Otolaryngology-Head and Neck Surgery, University of Rochester Medical Center, Box 629, 601 Elmwood Avenue, Rochester, NY 14642, USA
E-mail address: Matthew_miller@urmc.rochester.edu

Med Clin N Am 94 (2010) 1003–1015
doi:10.1016/j.mcna.2010.05.001
0025-7125/10/$ – see front matter © 2010 Elsevier Inc. All rights reserved.

medical.theclinics.com

development of new nodules.[7,8] The gestational effects are most pronounced in the third trimester and in the first 3 months postpartum[7] and are likely secondary to the effects of estrogens and progesterone. These hormones may also be responsible for the observed association between uterine fibroids and thyroid nodules.[9]

EPIDEMIOLOGY OF THYROID NODULES

The point prevalence of thyroid nodules is variably reported throughout the literature. This rate has been dependent on the population studied, the detection method, and the definition used. Among large and heterogeneous populations, palpable nodules are present in 0.2% to 21% and may be more common in women and older patients.[3,10–14] Palpation is generally considered to be the least sensitive and specific means of detection and is thought to be unreliable for nodules smaller than 1 cm.[11] Physical examination of the thyroid, however, is inexpensive, is not technically demanding, and is easily performed in just about any clinical setting. Consequently, it is advised that any head and neck examination include palpation of the gland to evaluate for nodules or thyromegaly. The presence of a palpable thyroid nodule should lead the clinician to obtain follow-up testing, which typically includes thyroid ultrasound.

Ultrasound has the benefit of being a more sensitive test than physical examination for the detection of thyroid nodules. It is estimated that palpation alone fails to detect up to two thirds of sonographically identifiable nodules.[3,11] Not surprisingly, prevalence rates for thyroid nodules are significantly higher when ultrasound is used as the screening modality. Among large series of asymptomatic patients, 19% to 35% have solitary or multiple nodules on ultrasound.[3,10–13] With high-resolution (ie, 13 MHz) techniques, this number approaches 70%.[14]

Histopathologic examination remains the gold standard for evaluation of thyroid nodules and, consequently, autopsy studies likely provide the most accurate representation of prevalence. Although the sample preparation techniques and definitions of nodules are somewhat variable, most autopsy studies have found nodular thyroid disease in 50% to 65% of patients.[10]

WHICH NODULES ARE CLINICALLY RELEVANT?

We have established that thyroid nodules are common and that there may be a set of clinical features that predispose patients to them. The previously mentioned prevalence rates should be interpreted with caution, however, because a large proportion of the nodules identified in these series were smaller than 1 cm. Consensus guidelines from a variety of professional societies have suggested that 1 cm be the threshold of significance for most nodules.[1,5,15,16]

An argument against the comprehensive evaluation of subcentimeter nodules stems from an understanding of the natural history of well-differentiated (for the most part papillary) carcinomas smaller than 1 cm (ie, microcarcinomas). Papillary thyroid microcarcinoma has been found incidentally on 2% to 36% of autopsies, suggesting that it may not be a clinically relevant finding in a number of individuals.[17–20] Furthermore, there has been no established survival benefit to identifying, or in some cases treating, papillary thyroid microcarcinoma.[5,20,21] Given that papillary thyroid microcarcinoma has a generally benign course, identification of these lesions may result in a patient being subject to potentially unnecessary surgery. Despite all of these factors, some subcentimeter nodules may indeed warrant further diagnostic evaluation. Indications for the detailed work-up of subcentimeter nodules are discussed later.

Another driving force behind the consensus guidelines stems from the inaccuracy of fine-needle aspiration (FNA) biopsy among subcentimeter nodules. FNA is considered to be the principal diagnostic tool in the evaluation of thyroid nodules. It has been shown that specimen adequacy rates, sensitivity, and negative predictive value of FNA are all reduced among nodules measuring 10 mm or less. These effects are most pronounced when the nodule is smaller than 5 mm.[22,23]

THE THYROID INCIDENTALOMA

Similar to the subcentimeter nodules, thyroid incidentalomas may or may not be clinically relevant depending on the circumstances of their identification. A thyroid incidentaloma is defined as a nodule not previously suspected or clinically apparent, but discovered on a radiographic study.[5] Incidentalomas have been described in many clinical contexts. Not uncommonly, they are brought to light after carotid ultrasound. Steele and colleagues[24] found thyroid nodules in 9.4% of 168 patients undergoing carotid duplex sonography. Many were greater than 1 cm in size and nearly one third harbored carcinomas (Fig. 1). It has been argued that any patient with an incidentaloma discovered on ultrasound should undergo dedicated thyroid and lateral neck sonography.[5]

CT and MRI studies may also reveal occult nodular thyroid disease. Incidentalomas have been observed in 10% to 17% of CTs and MRIs performed for nonthyroid indications (Fig. 2).[25–27] Although approximately 10% of the nodules ultimately prove to be malignant, these modalities remain limited in their ability to differentiate benign from cancerous nodules.[25,26] The presence of calcifications, anteroposterior to transverse diameter ratio greater than 1, and attenuation greater than 130 Hounsfield units on CT have been associated with an increased risk of carcinoma in one retrospective review.[25] No definitive criteria have been established, however, and it is recommended that CT incidentalomas be followed-up by formal thyroid ultrasound and possibly FNA.[5,25–27]

As positron emission tomography scanning has become more popular in recent years, it has also become a more frequent means of detecting thyroid incidentalomas (Fig. 3). Although large studies have found that only 1% to 2% of patients demonstrate ^{18}F-fluorodeoxyglucose uptake in the thyroid,[28–30] the malignancy rates are high.

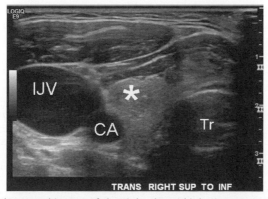

Fig. 1. Transverse ultrasound image of the right thyroid lobe in a patient who was incidentally discovered to have a 2-cm thyroid nodule (*asterisk*) during carotid duplex scanning. Visible are the trachea (Tr), internal jugular vein (IJV), and common carotid artery (CA).

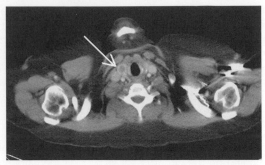

Fig. 2. Axial CT scan demonstrating an incidentally discovered nodule in the right thyroid lobe (*arrow*). Ultrasound-guided FNA biopsy revealed evidence of a follicular neoplasm.

Twenty-six percent to 67% of thyroid glands with focal ^{18}F-fluorodeoxyglucose avidity are ultimately found to contain carcinoma. This does not hold true for glands with diffuse ^{18}F-fluorodeoxyglucose uptake.[29–31] Consequently, it has been recommended that any patient with evidence of a focal increase in ^{18}F-fluorodeoxyglucose uptake undergo further evaluation.[1,5]

DIAGNOSTIC APPROACH

Ultrasound and FNA biopsy each play a prominent role in the evaluation of clinically or incidentally discovered thyroid nodules. Indeed, ultrasound and FNA are critical points in any management algorithm. Other historical, physical examination, imaging, and laboratory findings, however, also interplay with these studies. Ultimately, each of these elements assist in the further stratification of patients with nodules into lower- and higher-risk groups for thyroid carcinoma and should guide the decision between continued medical management and surgical referral.

IMPORTANT HISTORICAL ELEMENTS

Several components of a patient's medical, family, and social history may be germane to the evaluation of their thyroid nodule. The most important of these seems to be exposure to ionizing radiation. Patients exposed to radiation, particularly in childhood, are among the highest-risk groups for the development of thyroid carcinoma.[5,32–35] The latency period between exposure and development of carcinoma may be

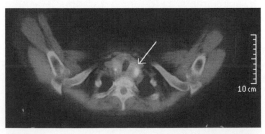

Fig. 3. ^{18}F-fluorodeoxyglucose positron emission tomography/CT fusion image of a patient who was being treated for a head and neck squamous cell carcinoma. This incidentally discovered left-sided nodule (*arrow*) was found on FNA to contain papillary thyroid carcinoma.

decades long, reaching its peak between 25 and 30 years after exposure.[35] A history of childhood malignancy, particularly Hodgkin's and non-Hodgkin's lymphoma, also increases the relative risk of thyroid carcinoma by a factor of approximately 3.5 times in a manner that seems to be independent of radiation therapy.[33]

Another historical risk factor to explore is a patient's family history. A single parent with a history of papillary thyroid carcinoma increases a patient's risk by a factor of three to five times.[36,37] The risk exceeds six times when the index patient has a sibling with papillary cancer.[36] In the context of medullary carcinoma, the increase in familial risk is staggering, with standardized incidence ratios in excess of 4000 for children of affected parents.[37] Other familial disorders, such as Cowden syndrome, Carney complex, familial polyposis, and the multiple endocrine neoplasia type 2 syndromes, are associated with increased risk for thyroid cancer and should prompt detailed evaluation in affected individuals who present with nodules.[1] Age at presentation also seems to have an effect; patients less than 45 years old are significantly more likely to have malignancy in the presence of a thyroid nodule.[38]

When observed in the presence of a nodule, hoarseness may also be an indicator of malignancy. Randolph and Kamani[39] found that this complaint, although not highly sensitive, was very specific in the preoperative identification of patients with invasive thyroid carcinoma. When coupled with laryngoscopy and confirmation of vocal fold paresis, the sensitivity and specificity were 75% and 100%, respectively. Raza and colleagues[38] found a similar relationship between vocal fold immobility and the presence of carcinoma. These studies help underscore the importance of vocal fold evaluation in the context of thyroid disease, particularly among those patients scheduled to undergo thyroidectomy.

DIAGNOSTIC STUDIES

All patients with known or suspected thyroid nodules should undergo testing for thyrotropin levels, also known as "thyroid-stimulating hormone" (TSH). The risk of malignancy in a thyroid nodule has been shown to be significantly greater in patients with elevated TSH.[40–42] Patients with a nodule and concomitant hypothyroidism have an adjusted odds ratio of malignancy in excess of 11.[41] Moreover, the risk of carcinoma seems to increase incrementally within the range of normal TSH values.[40,41] Interestingly, when compared with euthyroid and hypothyroid patients, individuals with low serum TSH have a reduced risk of carcinoma that is highly statistically significant.[42] As a result, a number of societies now recommend that serum TSH levels be drawn at the time a nodule is identified.[1,5,15,16] The presence of an elevated or normal TSH in the context of a nodule should prompt further testing to rule-out carcinoma. If the TSH is low, however, scintigraphy is the most appropriate next step. In the context of subclinical or overt hyperthyroidism, a "cold" nodule may still represent a thyroid carcinoma and a biopsy should be obtained. Conversely, autonomously functioning (ie, "hot") nodules on ^{123}I or pertechnetate scans are almost universally benign and do not warrant additional testing.[43,44]

One additional study that merits mentioning is calcitonin. Calcitonin is a sensitive and specific tumor marker used in the diagnosis, surveillance, and prognosis of medullary thyroid carcinoma (MTCA).[45] In the context of a family history of medullary carcinoma or multiple endocrine neoplasia syndromes, the presence of a nodule should alert the examiner to the possibility of MTCA. If not already performed, genetic testing for RET proto-oncogene and serum calcitonin levels should be obtained in this scenario.[45] Patients with the familial type represent a minority of MTCA patients and are likely to be identified on the basis of their family history and stigmata of the associated syndromes. Sporadic cases of MTCA are more common, but may be less clinically apparent. These patients are generally not distinguishable from any other individual presenting with a thyroid nodule and are managed in the usual fashion. Unfortunately, FNA may be less reliable in the context of MTCA: there is a considerable amount of overlap of cytologic features with other tumors[46] and the sensitivity for detecting MTCA is low in some series.[47] In response to these issues, Hahm and colleagues[47] explored the role that calcitonin might play in ruling out MTCA. Their work demonstrated that only 1% of normal controls had serum calcitonin levels above 10 pg/mL. Likewise, they found that none of the MTCA patients had levels below 10 pg/mL and that each of them had levels in excess of 100 pg/mL after pentagastrin stimulation. This was true for both sporadic and familial MTCA.[47] These and similar results have led many to suggest that calcitonin screening is an essential and cost-effective component of the diagnostic algorithm for thyroid nodules.[47,48] This recommendation has yet to gain widespread acceptance.

THYROID ULTRASOUND

Once a patient with a known or suspected nodule has had a complete history, physical examination, and serum TSH level completed, the next step in their evaluation should include sonographic evaluation of the thyroid and lateral neck compartments.[1,5,15,16] Ultrasound is the most sensitive and specific radiographic detection method for thyroid nodules. It allows for the confirmation and further characterization of both palpable nodules and incidentalomas. It has been the most widely studied imaging modality in the context of nodular thyroid disease. The literature has provided countless examples of sonographic features associated with an increased risk for malignancy. Among the most robustly predictive parameters are microcalcifications, size greater than 4 cm, hypoechogenicity, solid nodules, intranodular vascularization, irregular or microlobulated borders, length/width ratio greater than one, and the presence of solitary versus multiple nodules.[49–54] One additional feature worth noting is the presence of nodal disease within the lateral compartments of the neck. The presence of lymph nodes greater than 1 cm may be indicative of carcinoma and may portend a worse prognosis in patients with microcarcinoma.[5,21]

Although no single sonographic finding is diagnostic, combinations of these are known to be of high sensitivity and specificity for carcinoma[53] and are indications for FNA biopsy. Likewise, in the proper clinical context, the presence of any one of these characteristics may raise suspicion for thyroid cancer and prompt the clinician to obtain a biopsy.

FNA BIOPSY

FNA is the most cost-effective and accurate means of evaluating thyroid nodules.[1] It is generally recommended that FNA be performed for essentially any nodule greater than or equal to 1 cm.[1,5,15,16] The Society of Radiologists in Ultrasound have somewhat more stringent criteria, recommending FNA for 1-cm nodules only if microcalcifications are present.[55] Subcentimeter nodules may also be considered for biopsy if the patient has high-risk characteristics in their medical or family history (as noted previously); suspicious sonographic features; enlarged lymph nodes in the lateral compartment (again pointing to the importance of evaluating the entire neck during sonography for thyroid nodules); or vocal fold paralysis.[1,5,16,21,22] Nodules smaller than 5 mm should generally not be considered for biopsy, however, because of the low sensitivity and accuracy of diagnosis for these lesions.[1,22,23]

In the context of a palpable nodule, FNA may be performed with or without ultrasound guidance. The ultrasound-guided technique has been advocated as a means to improve needle placement and diagnostic yield during FNA, even among palpable disease. Ultrasound-guided FNA has been shown to reduce the number of false-negative biopsies performed[5,56] for solitary nodules and, in the context of multinodular goiter, it allows for more accurate sampling of a dominant or suspicious nodule.[57] Ultrasound guidance is considered the procedure of choice for all nonpalpable, cystic, and posteriorly placed nodules[1] and, in the author's opinion, any palpable nodule. Regardless of whether ultrasound is used, on-site evaluation by a cytopathology professional is desirable. Although the diagnosis may not always be rendered, the specimen can be examined for adequacy. This step is vital to reducing the number of nondiagnostic results and repeated aspirations.[58]

FOLLOW-UP AND SURGICAL REFERRAL

The decision to refer for surgical evaluation depends to a great extent on the interpretation of the FNA. Reporting of FNA cytology varies between institutions and depends on the training and classification system used by the cytopathologist. Although the nomenclature may differ slightly, cytopathologists generally render their diagnoses within one of the following broad categories: nondiagnostic or inadequate, benign, cellular follicular lesion, follicular neoplasm, suspicious for malignancy, or malignant.[59] Inadequate samples should prompt rebiopsy (with ultrasound guidance if not used initially). Multiple nondiagnostic FNAs may be observed or referred to surgery.[1] Biopsies found to be benign on FNA have a very small probability of harboring carcinoma. Between 1% and 11% of lesions called benign on FNA ultimately prove to be malignancies.[16,60,61] These nodules may be followed with serial ultrasound examinations every 6 to 18 months.[1] If clinical or sonographic features change, it may be reasonable to perform a repeat biopsy. If a second or third FNA results in a benign diagnosis, however, the likelihood of malignancy is minimal and either medical therapy or expectant management is appropriate.[60,62,63] Benign solid nodules have been treated successfully using levothyroxine suppression, ethanol sclerosis, or percutaneous laser ablation.[63–65] Recurrent cysts may either be removed surgically or treated with ethanol sclerotherapy.[1]

Cellular follicular lesions carry an approximately 5% to 20% risk of malignancy.[16,59] The decision to refer to surgery in this group relies heavily on clinical suspicion for carcinoma. High-risk factors for cancer include age greater than 60 years, male gender, size greater than 4 cm, rapid growth, rock-hard texture of the nodule, vocal cord paralysis, previous exposure to radiation, family history of thyroid cancer, and growth during adequate thyroxine suppression.[59] The presence of any of these factors in the presence of a cellular follicular lesion is an indication for surgery.[1,15] Alternatively, if these risk factors are not present, a repeat ultrasound with or without rebiopsy may be performed in 6 to 18 months.

Follicular neoplasia is a more worrisome finding. Approximately 25% to 30% of follicular neoplasms are malignant on permanent histopathologic sectioning.[16,66,67] The rate approaches 45% in the presence of cytologic atypia.[68] Patients with these lesions should be referred for surgery. Likewise, the "suspicious for malignancy" category carries with it a 50% to 75% risk of cancer. These patients also should be referred to the surgeon. FNA diagnostic of malignancy should also be referred for surgical thyroidectomy. Repeat biopsy is not generally used because the false-positive rate is less than 2% in most series (**Fig. 4**).[61]

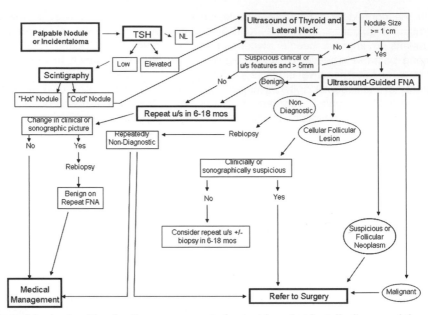

Fig. 4. A basic algorithm for the management of palpable or incidentally discovered thyroid nodules. Please refer to the text for more detailed recommendations regarding management and follow-up. FNA, fine-needle aspiration; NL, normal; TSH, thyroid-stimulating hormone.

The specifics of surgical management are often the subject of controversy and are beyond the scope of this article. In general, patients with suspicious lesions should undergo at least thyroid lobectomy and isthmusectomy, with completion thyroidectomy reserved for histopathologic confirmation of malignancy on frozen or permanent section. Patients with confirmed malignant disease by FNA should undergo total thyroidectomy with nodal dissection of the at-risk or involved neck compartments.[1,15]

Recently, a number of new technologies have been introduced into the arena of thyroid surgery. Advances in endoscopic, minimally invasive, and robotic techniques have allowed thyroidectomy to be performed through smaller and more cosmetically appealing incisions.[69–71] These approaches have been touted as being less invasive and less prone to complications. The only variables that have definitive benefits with respect to complication rates of thyroid surgery, however, are the experience and volume of individual surgeons and hospitals.[72] This underscores the importance of referral to centers and surgeons that frequently perform thyroidectomy.

Regardless of technique, the most worrisome complications of thyroidectomy include recurrent laryngeal nerve injury and, in the case of total thyroidectomy, hypocalcemia. Iatrogenic nerve injury is thought to occur in approximately 1% of cases. The risk may be reduced by the use of intraoperative nerve monitoring.[73] Permanent hypoparathyroidism and subsequent hypocalcemia is observed in approximately 0.4% to 13% of patients undergoing total thyroidectomy.[74] Close monitoring and, when necessary, replacement of serum calcium in the postoperative period are essential.

FUTURE DIRECTIONS

When one considers the fact that a significant number of patients with "suspicious" cytology and an even larger proportion of those with "follicular" lesions undergo thyroidectomy for benign disease, it is apparent that FNA may not be a specific enough test in some contexts. To combat this, much attention has been paid to molecular characterization of FNA biopsy specimens. Several genetic mutations have been identified that are specific to papillary or follicular carcinoma. These mutations (*BRAF, RET/PTC, RAS*, and *PAX8/PPAR$_\gamma$*) have been identified in preoperative FNA specimens by Nikiforov and colleagues.[75] In their series of 470 FNA samples, 97% of mutation-positive nodules were found to be malignant on permanent histologic sectioning. The authors concluded that testing for these mutations improved the accuracy of FNA when used in a complementary fashion. Other studies have used galectin-3,[76] BRAF,[77] and transcriptional profiles (ie, microarrays)[78] as adjuncts to FNA. Unfortunately, these tests are not widely available and are not sufficiently sensitive or specific for the diagnosis of carcinoma. They remain investigational at this point, but may in time become standard adjuncts to or even replacements for FNA cytology.

SUMMARY

Thyroid nodules are common occurrences. Although they are often palpable, many are discovered incidentally during unrelated radiographic studies. All patients with nodular thyroid disease should undergo serum TSH testing and, if euthyroid or hypothyroid, dedicated thyroid and lateral neck ultrasound. FNA biopsy should be performed on all nodules greater than 1 cm, all positron emission tomography incidentalomas, and all nodules 5 mm or larger in patients with high-risk clinical or sonographic features. Suspicious or frankly malignant cytology on FNA biopsy should prompt referral to a surgeon with expertise in thyroidectomy.

REFERENCES

1. Cooper DS, Doherty GM, Haugen BR, et al. Revised American Thyroid Association Management guidelines for patients with thyroid nodules and differentiated thyroid cancer. Thyroid 2009;19(11):1167–214.
2. Knudsen K, Laurberg P, Perrild H, et al. Risk factors for goiter and thyroid nodules. Thyroid 2002;12(10):879–88.
3. Ezzat S, Sarti DA, Cain DR, et al. Thyroid incidentalomas: prevalence by palpation and ultrasonography. Arch Intern Med 1994;154:1838–40.
4. Galanti MR, Granath F, Cnattingius S, et al. Cigarette smoking and the risk of goitre and thyroid nodules amongst parous women. J Intern Med 2005;258(3): 257–64.
5. Cibas ES, Alexander EK, Benson CB, et al. Indications for thyroid FNA and pre-FNA requirements: a synopsis of the National Cancer Institute Thyroid Fine-Needle Aspiration State of the Science Conference. Diagn Cytopathol 2008; 36(6):390–9.
6. Antonelli A, Silvano G, Bianchi F, et al. Risk of thyroid nodules in subjects occupationally exposed to radiation: a cross sectional study. Occup Environ Med 1995;52(8):500–4.
7. Kung AW, Chau MT, Lao TT, et al. The effect of pregnancy on thyroid nodule formation. J Clin Endocrinol Metab 2002;87(3):1010–4.
8. Struve CW, Haupt S, Ohlen S. Influence of frequency of previous pregnancies on the prevalence of thyroid nodules in women without clinical evidence of thyroid disease. Thyroid 1993;3(1):7–10.

9. Spinos N, Terzis G, Crysanthopoulou A, et al. Increased frequency of thyroid nodules and breast fibroadenomas in women with uterine fibroids. Thyroid 2007;17(12):1257–9.
10. Wang C, Crapo LM. The epidemiology of thyroid disease and implications for screening. Endocrinol Metab Clin North Am 1997;26(1):189–218.
11. Tan GH, Gharib H, Reading CC. Solitary thyroid nodule: comparison between palpation and ultrasonography. Arch Intern Med 1995;155:2418–23.
12. Brander A, Viikinkoski P, Nickels J, et al. Thyroid gland: US screening in a random adult population. Radiology 1991;181:683–7.
13. Brander A, Viikinkoski P, Nickels J, et al. Thyroid gland: US screening in middle-aged women with no previous thyroid disease. Radiology 1989;173:507–10.
14. Guth S, Theune U, Aberle J, et al. Very high prevalence of thyroid nodules detected by high frequency (13 MHz) ultrasound examination. Eur J Clin Invest 2009;39(8):699–706.
15. Gharib H, Papini E, Valcavi R, et al. American Association of Clinical Endocrinologists and Associazione Medici Endocrinologi medical guidelines for clinical practice for the diagnosis and management of thyroid nodules. Endocr Pract 2006;12(1):63–102.
16. Baloch ZW, Cibas ES, Clark DP, et al. The National Cancer Institute thyroid fine needle aspiration state of the science conference: a summation. Cytojournal 2008;5(6):1–17.
17. Kovacs GL, Ganda G, Vadasz G, et al. Epidemiology of thyroid microcarcinoma found in autopsy series found in areas of different iodine uptake. Thyroid 2005; 15(2):152–7.
18. de Matos PS, Ferreira AP, Ward LS. Prevalence of papillary microcarcinoma of the thyroid in Brazilian autopsy and surgical series. Endocr Pathol 2006;17(2):165–73.
19. Yamamoto Y, Maeda T, Izumi K, et al. Occult papillary carcinoma of the thyroid. A study of 408 autopsy cases. Cancer 1990;65(5):1173–9.
20. Pazaitou-Panayiotou K, Capezzone M, Pacini F. Clinical features and therapeutic implication of papillary thyroid microcarcinoma. Thyroid 2007;17(11):1085–92.
21. Sugitani I, Toda K, Yamada K, et al. Three distinctly different kinds of papillary thyroid microcarcinoma should be recognized: our treatment strategies and outcomes. World J Surg 2010;34(6):1222–31.
22. Kim EW, Lee EJ, Kim SH, et al. Ultrasound-guided fine-needle aspiration biopsy of thyroid nodules: comparison of efficacy according to nodule size. Thyroid 2009;19(1):27–31.
23. Leenhardt L, Hejblum G, Franc B, et al. Indications and limits of ultrasound-guided cytology in the management of non-palpable thyroid nodules. J Clin Endocrinol Metab 1999;84:24–8.
24. Steele SR, Martin MJ, Mullenix PS, et al. The significance of incidental thyroid abnormalities identified during carotid duplex ultrasonography. Arch Surg 2005;140:981–5.
25. Yoon DW, Chang SK, Choi CS, et al. The prevalence and significance of incidental thyroid nodules identified on computed tomography. J Comput Assist Tomogr 2008;32:810–5.
26. Shetty SK, Maher MM, Hahn PF, et al. Significance of incidental thyroid lesions detected on CT: correlation among CT, sonography, and pathology. AJR Am J Roentgenol 2006;187:1349–56.
27. Yousem DM, Huang T, Loevner LA, et al. Clinical and economic impact of incidental thyroid lesions found with CT and MR. AJNR Am J Neuroradiol 1997;18: 1423–8.

28. Chen YK, Ding HJ, Chen KT, et al. Prevalence and risk of cancer of focal thyroid incidentaloma identified by 18F-fluorodeoxyglucose positron emission tomography for cancer screening in healthy subjects. Anticancer Res 2005;25(2B):1421–6.
29. Kim TY, Kim WB, Ryu JS, et al. 18F-Fluorodeoxyglucose uptake in thyroid from positron emission tomogram (PET) for evaluation in cancer patients: high prevalence of malignancy in thyroid PET incidentaloma. Laryngoscope 2005;115:1074–8.
30. Shie P, Cardarelli R, Sprawls K, et al. Systematic review: prevalence of malignant incidental thyroid nodules identified on fluorine-18 fluorodeoxyglucose positron emission tomography. Nucl Med Commun 2009;30(9):742–8.
31. Liu Y. Clinical significance of thyroid uptake on F18-fl uorodeoxyglucose positron emission tomography. Ann Nucl Med 2009;23:17–23.
32. Dal Maso L, Boselli C, La Vecchia C, et al. Risk factors for thyroid cancer: an epidemiological review focused on nutritional factors. Cancer Causes Control 2009;20(1):75–86.
33. Taylor AJ, Croft AP, Palace AM, et al. Risk of thyroid cancer in survivors of childhood cancer: results from the British Childhood Cancer Survivor Study. Int J Cancer 2009;125(10):2400–5.
34. Perrier ND, Ituarte P, Siperstein AE, et al. Latency period of thyroid neoplasia after radiation exposure. Ann Surg 2004;239(4):536–43.
35. Schneider AB, Ron E, Lubin J, et al. Dose-response relationships for radiation-induced thyroid cancer and thyroid nodules: evidence for the prolonged effects of radiation on the thyroid. J Clin Endocrinol Metab 1993;77(2):362–9.
36. Hemminki K, Eng C, Chen B. Familial risks for nonmedullary thyroid cancer. J Clin Endocrinol Metab 2005;90(10):5747–53.
37. Hemminki K, Dong C. Familial relationships in thyroid cancer by histopathological type. Int J Cancer 2000;85(2):201–5.
38. Raza SN, Shah MD, Palme CE, et al. Risk factors for well-differentiated thyroid carcinoma in patients with thyroid nodular disease. Otolaryngol Head Neck Surg 2008;139(1):21–6.
39. Randolph GW, Kamani D. The importance of preoperative laryngoscopy in patients undergoing thyroidectomy: voice, vocal cord function, and the preoperative detection of invasive thyroid malignancy. Surgery 2006;139:357–62.
40. Polyzos SA, Kita M, Efstathiadou Z, et al. Serum thyrotropin concentration as a biochemical predictor of thyroid malignancy in patients presenting with thyroid nodules. J Cancer Res Clin Oncol 2008;134(9):953–60.
41. Boelaert K, Horacek J, Holder RL, et al. Serum thyrotropin concentration as a novel predictor of malignancy in thyroid nodules investigated by fine-needle aspiration. J Clin Endocrinol Metab 2006;91(11):4295–301.
42. Fiore E, Rago T, Provenzale MA, et al. Lower levels of TSH are associated with a lower risk of papillary thyroid cancer in patients with thyroid nodular disease: thyroid autonomy may play a protective role. Endocr Relat Cancer 2009;16(4):1251–60.
43. Meller J, Becker W. The continuing importance of thyroid scintigraphy in the era of high-resolution ultrasound. Eur J Nucl Med 2002;29(Suppl 2):S425–38.
44. Wilhelm SM. Utility of I-123 thyroid uptake scan in incidental thyroid nodules: an old test with a new role. Surgery 2008;144(4):511–5.
45. Jimenez C, Hu MI, Gagel RF. Management of medullary thyroid carcinoma. Endocrinol Metab Clin North Am 2008;37:481–96.
46. Forrest CH, Frost FA, de Boer WB, et al. Medullary carcinoma of the thyroid: accuracy of diagnosis by fine-needle aspiration cytology. Cancer Cytopathol 1998;84:295–302.

47. Hahm JR, Lee MS, Min YK, et al. Routine measurement of serum calcitonin is useful for early detection of medullary thyroid carcinoma in patients with nodular thyroid diseases. Thyroid 2001;11(1):73–80.
48. Cheung K, Roman SA, Wang TS, et al. Calcitonin measurement in the evaluation of thyroid nodules in the United States: a cost-effectiveness and decision analysis. J Clin Endocrinol Metab 2008;93(6):2173–80.
49. Wang N, Xu Y, Ge C, et al. Association of sonographically detected calcification with thyroid carcinoma. Head Neck 2006;28(12):1077–83.
50. Frates MC, Benson CB, Doubilet PM, et al. Prevalence and distribution of carcinoma in patients with solitary and multiple thyroid nodules on sonography. J Clin Endocrinol Metab 2006;91(9):3411–7.
51. Tae HJ, Lim DJ, Baek KH, et al. Diagnostic value of ultrasonography to distinguish between benign and malignant lesions in the management of thyroid nodules. Thyroid 2007;17(5):461–6.
52. Alexander EK, Marqusee E, Orcutt J, et al. Thyroid nodule shape and prediction of malignancy. Thyroid 2004;14(11):953–8.
53. Ahn SS, Kim EK, Kang DR, et al. Biopsy of thyroid nodules: comparison of three sets of guidelines. AJR Am J Roentgenol 2010;194(1):31–7.
54. McCoy KL, Jabbour N, Ogilvie JB, et al. The incidence of cancer and rate of false-negative cytology in thyroid nodules greater than or equal to 4 cm in size. Surgery 2007;142(6):837–44.
55. Frates MC, Benson CB, Charboneau JW, et al. Management of thyroid nodules detected at US: Society of Radiologists in Ultrasound consensus conference statement. Radiology 2005;237(3):794–800.
56. Pitman MB, Abele J, Ali SZ, et al. Techniques for thyroid FNA: a synopsis of the National Cancer Institute Thyroid Fine-Needle Aspiration State of the Science Conference. Diagn Cytopathol 2008;36(6):407–24.
57. Gandolfi PP, Frisina A, Raffa M, et al. The incidence of thyroid carcinoma in multinodular goiter: retrospective analysis. Acta Biomed 2004;75:114–7.
58. Zhu W, Michael CW. How important is on-site adequacy assessment for thyroid FNA? An evaluation of 883 cases. Diagn Cytopathol 2007;35(3):183–6.
59. Guidelines of the Papanicolaou Society of Cytopathology for the examination of fine-needle aspiration specimens from thyroid nodules. The Papanicolaou Society of Cytopathology Task Force on Standards of Practice. Diagn Cytopathol 1996;15(1):84–9.
60. Oertel YC, Felipe LM, Mendoza MG, et al. Value of repeated fine needle aspirations of the thyroid: an analysis of over ten thousand FNAs. Thyroid 2007;17(11):1061–6.
61. Yang J, Schnadig V, Logrono R, et al. Fine-needle aspiration of thyroid nodules: a study of 4703 patients with histologic and clinical correlations. Cancer Cytopathol 2007;111:306–15.
62. Orlandi A, Puscar A, Capriata E, et al. Repeated fine-needle aspiration of the thyroid in benign nodular thyroid disease: critical evaluation of long-term follow up. Thyroid 2005;15(3):274–8.
63. Sdano MT, Falciglia M, Welge JA, et al. Efficacy of thyroid hormone suppression for benign thyroid nodules: meta-analysis of randomized trials. Otolaryngol Head Neck Surg 2005;133:391–6.
64. Bennedbaek FN, Nielsen LK, Hegedüs L. Effect of percutaneous ethanol injection therapy versus suppressive doses of L-thyroxine on benign solitary solid cold thyroid nodules: a randomized trial. J Clin Endocrinol Metab 1998;83(3):830–5.

65. Papini E, Guglielmi R, Bizzarri G, et al. Treatment of benign cold nodules: a randomized clinical trial of percutaneous laser ablation versus levothyroixine therapy or follow-up. Thyroid 2007;17(3):229–35.
66. Mihai R, Parker AJ, Roskell D, et al. One in four patients with follicular thyroid cytology (THY3) has a thyroid carcinoma. Thyroid 2009;19(1):33–7.
67. Raparia K, Min SK, Mody DR, et al. Clinical outcomes for "suspicious" category in thyroid fine-needle aspiration biopsy: patient's sex and nodule size are possible predictors of malignancy. Arch Pathol Lab Med 2009;133(5):787–90.
68. Goldstein RE, Netterville JL, Burkey B, et al. Implications of follicular neoplasms, atypia, and lesions suspicious for malignancy diagnosed by fine-needle aspiration of thyroid nodules. Ann Surg 2002;235(5):656–62.
69. Gal I, Solymosi T, Szabo Z, et al. Minimally invasive video-assisted thyroidectomy and conventional thyroidectomy: a prospective randomized study. Surg Endosc 2008;22:2445–9.
70. Cavicchi O, Piccin O, Ceroni AR, et al. Minimally invasive nonendoscopic thyroidectomy. Otolaryngol Head Neck Surg 2006;135(5):744–7.
71. Kang SW, Lee SC, Lee SH, et al. Robotic thyroid surgery using a gasless, transaxillary approach and the da Vinci S system: the operative outcomes of 338 consecutive patients. Surgery 2009;146(6):1048–55.
72. Sosa JA, Bowman HM, Tielsch JM, et al. The importance of surgeon experience for clinical and economic outcomes from thyroidectomy. Ann Surg 1998;228(3).320–30.
73. Miller MC, Spiegel JR. Identification and monitoring of the recurrent laryngeal nerve during thyroidectomy. Surg Oncol Clin N Am 2008;17(1):121–44.
74. Fewins J, Simpson CB, Miller FR. Complications of thyroid and parathyroid surgery. Otolaryngol Clin North Am 2003;36:189–206.
75. Nikiforov YE, Steward DL, Robinson-Smith TM, et al. Molecular testing for mutations in improving the fine-needle aspiration diagnosis of thyroid nodules. J Clin Endocrinol Metab 2009;94(6):2092–8.
76. Bartolazzi A, Orlandi F, Saggiorato E, et al. Galectin-3-expression analysis in the surgical selection of follicular thyroid nodules with indeterminate fine-needle aspiration cytology: a prospective multicentre study. Lancet Oncol 2008;9(6):543–9.
77. Bentz BG, Miller BT, Holden JA, et al. B-RAF V600E mutational analysis of fine needle aspirates correlates with diagnosis of thyroid nodules. Otolaryngol Head Neck Surg 2009;140:709–14.
78. Lubitz CC, Ugrass SK, Kazam JJ, et al. Microarray analysis of thyroid fine-needle aspirates accurately classifies benign and malignant lesions. J Mol Diagn 2006;8:490–8.

Evaluating the Adult Patient with a Neck Mass

Tara L. Rosenberg, MD[a], Jimmy J. Brown, MD, DDS[b],
Gina D. Jefferson, MD[a],*

KEYWORDS

• Neck mass • Adult • Differential diagnosis
• Cervical lymphadenopathy

The internist frequently encounters adult patients with a neck mass. The objective of this article is to provide the internist with general considerations when confronted with an adult patient presenting with a neck mass. A thorough gathering of historical information and a complete physical examination are crucial in refining a differential diagnosis for these patients. The location of the mass, details surrounding its appearance, and overall time course are important factors to help differentiate neoplastic disease from other possibilities in the long differential diagnosis. A persistent neck mass in an adult older than 40 years should raise a suspicion of malignancy. A neck mass in a young adult patient is more likely to be an inflammatory, congenital, or traumatic process. The clinical evaluation of a persistent neck mass may also require imaging studies or biopsy to establish the diagnosis.

Of particular concern is the adult patient who is treated with antibiotics but in whom the neck mass persists. Patients 40 years and older presenting with a neck mass have a high likelihood of harboring a malignant neoplasm. Neck mass persistence, progressive enlargement, or any other concern for a neoplastic process warrants referral to an otolaryngologist or other head and neck surgeon for further evaluation.

ANATOMIC CONSIDERATIONS

In addition to the patient's age, the location of a neck mass plays a key role in the formation of a differential diagnosis. The neck is divided into cervical triangles, and these triangles all have a common boundary, the sternocleidomastoid muscle. The posterior cervical triangle is bound anteriorly by the posterior aspect of the

[a] Department of Otolaryngology and Communicative Sciences, University of Mississippi Medical Center, 2500 North State Street, Jackson, MS 39126, USA
[b] Department of Otolaryngology – Head and Neck Surgery, Medical College of Georgia, 1120 Fifteenth Street, BP – 4109, Augusta, GA 30912, USA
* Corresponding author.
E-mail address: gjefferson@umc.edu

Med Clin N Am 94 (2010) 1017–1029
doi:10.1016/j.mcna.2010.05.007
0025-7125/10/$ – see front matter © 2010 Elsevier Inc. All rights reserved.

sternocleidomastoid muscle, posteriorly by the anterior border of the trapezius muscle, and inferiorly by the clavicle. The boundaries of the anterior cervical triangle are the median line of the neck, the inferior border of the mandible superiorly, and the anterior border of the sternocleidomastoid muscle posteriorly. The location of the neck mass in a particular lymphatic zone also provides the clinician a clue to the site of origin of a neoplastic or inflammatory process (**Fig. 1**A, B).

FINE-NEEDLE ASPIRATION

Fine-needle aspiration biopsy (FNAB) is the standard of care in working up an adult neck mass. FNAB, while highly dependent on the skill of the cytopathologist, is highly sensitive and specific for neoplasia, easily performed in the outpatient setting with local anesthesia, and may provide a specimen for Gram stain, acid-fast bacilli stain, or culture. In contrast to open biopsy, FNAB will not interfere with subsequent surgical treatment of a neoplastic condition. FNAB may also distinguish cystic from solid masses. While FNAB is an appropriate initial diagnostic procedure for a persistent neck mass, it should not be attempted on pulsatile neck masses. In general, FNAB is most safely performed after imaging studies are complete to avoid inadvertent biopsy of a vascular lesion.

IMAGING

In most situations, computed tomography (CT) of the neck with contrast is the best initial imaging study for evaluation of a neck mass in an adult. CT with contrast provides adequate information regarding, the size, extent, location, and characteristics of the mass. Cystic and solid lesions can be distinguished, and the relationship of the mass to other vital structures such as the airway, cranial nerves, and major blood vessels can be assessed. The scan will also reveal possible primary sites in the case of neoplastic disease. To encompass the entire upper aerodigestive tract, the ordering physician should request that the CT scan of the neck extend from the base of the skull to the thoracic inlet. If indicated, further imaging studies such as magnetic resonance imaging (MRI) can be obtained.[1]

MRI is an excellent imaging modality for soft tissue lesions, but is not required in most situations. MRI is more expensive and time consuming. However, MR imaging may be useful in certain clinical scenarios, for example, in the patient with iodine contrast reactions or for thyroid imaging. An example of an indication for MRI with contrast is the need to evaluate a thyroid mass that extends into the mediastinum. MRI is preferred in this clinical situation because the iodine load administered with CT scan is metabolized by the thyroid tissue and can interfere with radioactive iodine treatment.[1]

Ultrasound is the ideal imaging study for a thyroid lesion. This imaging modality, however, does not provide enough information about the character of a neck mass and the relationship to other structures for a routine evaluation of a neck mass outside of the central compartment. Therefore, if imaging is included in the workup, CT of the neck with contrast should be obtained.[2]

UPPER ENDOSCOPY

Occasionally the FNAB is diagnostic for carcinoma, yet no primary site can be identified on imaging or head and neck examination. This situation warrants a complete endoscopic examination of the upper aerodigestive tract under general anesthesia, with directed biopsies in an attempt to ascertain the primary site. Another indication for operating room management is for those cases where lymphoma is high in the

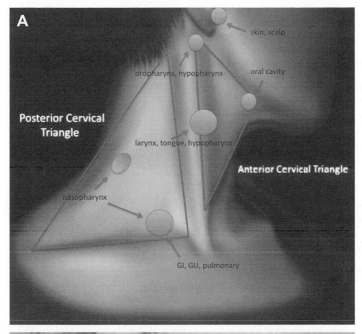

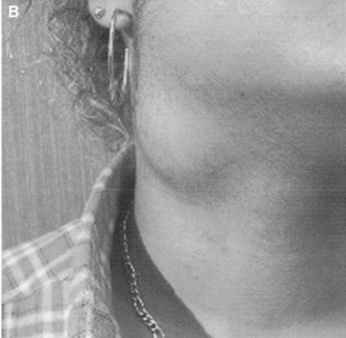

Fig. 1. (*A*) The major triangular divisions of the neck and lymphatic drainage patterns indicate primary location of inflammatory and neoplastic disease processes. GI, gastrointestinal; GU, genitourinary. (*B*) Adult patient with a neck mass located in the superior aspect of the anterior cervical triangle.

differential. A definitive diagnosis often requires an open neck biopsy to obtain sufficient amount of specimen to perform flow cytometry studies.

DIFFERENTIAL DIAGNOSIS OF NECK MASSES

The following sections are brief descriptions of pertinent historical information, physical examination findings, laboratory tests, and imaging studies for each differential diagnosis category. While not representing a complete list of differential diagnoses or diagnostic approach for an adult with a neck mass, the descriptions provide a framework on which to build clinical decision making. As illustrated in this article, the differential diagnosis is extensive and is easily remembered by employing the mnemonic "KITTENS" (**Table 1**) as initially described in Pasha's book, *Otolaryngology: Head and Neck Surgery Clinical Reference Guide*,[3] an acronym for **K**—congenital/developmental anomalies, **I**—infectious/inflammatory, **T**—trauma, **T**—toxic, **E**—endocrine, **N**—neoplasms, and **S**—systemic diseases.

K: Congenital/Developmental Anomalies

Thyroglossal duct cyst is the most common congenital neck anomaly and represents persistence of the thyroglossal duct. This cyst most commonly presents as a midline

Table 1 "KITTENS" mnemonic for the differential diagnosis of the adult neck mass	
K	**Congenital/developmental anomalies** Thyroglossal duct cyst Branchial cleft cyst Dermoid cyst Vascular malformation, ie, "lymphangioma," "lymphovenous malformation," etc
I	**Infectious/inflammatory** Lymphadenitis/cervical adenopathy Viral (EBV) Bacterial (cat scratch disease, mycobacteria, atypical mycobacteria)
T	**Trauma** Hematoma Pseudoaneurysm Laryngocele
T	**Toxic** Thyroid toxicosis
E	**Endocrine** Thyroid neoplasms Parathyroid neoplasms
N	**Neoplasms** Salivary gland Parapharyngeal space—salivary tumors, glomus tumors, neurogenic tumors Lipoma Lymphoma
S	**Systemic disease** Sarcoidosis Sjögren syndrome Kimura disease Castleman disease

Data from Pasha R. Otolaryngology: head and neck surgery clinical reference guide. 2nd edition. San Diego: Plural Publishing, Inc; 2006. p. 79, 207.

cystic mass, usually inferior to the hyoid bone that (classically at least) elevates with swallowing or protrusion of the tongue.[4] Thyroglossal duct cysts are usually diagnosed by the age of 5 years, and 60% of them are diagnosed before age 20. However, about 7% of the adult population still has this abnormality.[5] These cysts may become evident after an upper respiratory tract infection, and it is appropriate to treat any acutely infected thyroglossal cyst with antibiotics. An important consideration in adults is that this mass may contain, although rarely, the only functional thyroid tissue in the patient; therefore, palpation of a normal thyroid gland is a key aspect of the physical examination. CT scan of the neck with contrast is the single most important imaging study and should be obtained in adults with suspected thyroglossal duct cyst. The CT scan can confirm the presence of a thyroid gland. In addition, approximately 1% of adult thyroglossal duct cysts contain carcinoma foci, and CT scans can reveal calcifications in these areas of carcinoma.[4] Treatment involves complete excision.

Branchial cleft cysts are most commonly found in late childhood or early adulthood. Similar to thyroglossal duct cysts, they are frequently diagnosed following an upper respiratory tract infection when the mass becomes inflamed. Occasionally the mass resolves, but most often they persist as a soft mass in the neck. The first branchial cleft cyst is found at the mandibular angle inferior to the ear lobule along the inferior border of the mandible, and may have a tract that connects to the external auditory canal. The second branchial cleft cyst is the most common type, and may have a tract that opens along the anterior border of the sternocleidomastoid muscle. This cyst sometimes has a tract that opens in the oropharynx at the superior portion of the tonsillar fossa. CT of the neck with contrast is an appropriate imaging study in an adult patient. Initial management is with appropriate antibiotics if the mass is infected. Definitive treatment is complete surgical excision of the cyst and tract.[6]

Ranulas are mucus retention cysts or mucus extravasation pseudocysts in the floor of the mouth. A plunging ranula is a mucus extravasation pseudocyst that more commonly arises from the sublingual gland, and may present as a neck mass when it, by definition, extends through the mylohyoid muscle. History reveals a progressively enlarging cyst in the neck. A plunging ranula may present as a submandibular mass without obvious intraoral involvement, and waxes and wanes in size. Physical examination reveals a soft, compressible mass in the neck, usually in the submandibular triangle.[7] CT scan of the neck with contrast is the best imaging study to evaluate the mass.[3,8] Treatment is excision of the sublingual gland and ranula in continuity to minimize the risk of recurrence.[7]

Dermoid cysts are rare but may present as a painless, superficial, soft, doughy mass in the neck. The most common location in the neck is in the submental triangle (under the chin). Dermoid cysts most commonly present in children or young adults. The dermoid cyst progressively enlarges due to accumulation of sebaceous contents.[9] Some physicians advocate use of MRI to distinguish this mass from other neck masses,[10] but first-line evaluation for most neck masses in adults is CT of neck with contrast. Treatment is with surgical excision.

Lymphangioma, or lymphatic malformation, is a rare, congenital anomaly that usually presents in childhood and occasionally in adults. The majority of cases occur in the head and neck, mostly in the posterior triangle. Diagnosis is by history of a soft, compressible neck mass that usually enlarges proportionally with the growth of the patient. Characteristic findings of cyst-like structures on imaging studies like CT scan of the neck with contrast aid in diagnosis. Definitive diagnosis of lymphangioma is from operative pathology. Treatment regimens vary depending on macrocystic or microcystic features, but usually involve an attempt at complete surgical excision, although usually this is a difficult endeavor.[11]

I: Infectious/Inflammatory

Deep neck space infections and neck abscesses in adults are often caused by an odontogenic or salivary source. Other causes include penetrating trauma, spread of infection from more superficial infections, and in cases in which no source is identified, branchial cleft cysts or fistulae. Important historical information encompasses symptoms of infection including pain, swelling, erythema, fever, odontalgia and/or history of recent dental procedure, spontaneous purulent drainage, accompanied by a progressively enlarging neck mass. There may be airway compromise as well, depending on abscess size, specific neck location, and edema. Physical examination reveals a tender swelling in the neck with possible overlying erythema, induration, and local fluctuance. The imaging study of choice is a CT scan of the neck with contrast. Treatment involves appropriate antibiotics and surgical drainage depending on size and response to antibiotics.[12] An important point is that in adults, a necrotic, inflamed lymph node from a metastatic cancer may present in a similar manner to a neck abscess. If there is suspicion for a malignancy, CT of the neck will also be an important study (see N: neoplasms).

Acute sialadenitis presents with pain and swelling of the affected salivary gland, accompanied by systemic symptoms of infection. History taking should include onset of pain and swelling, gradual or rapid onset, odontalgia to assess for possible dental abscess, and medical and surgical history to identify risk factors. Common risk factors include an elderly, debilitated patient, dehydration, recent surgery, and recent dental procedures. Physical examination reveals local edema, erythema, induration, warmth, and tenderness to palpation, and likely reveals systemic signs of dehydration.[13] Palpate the involved area to assess for fluctuance that might indicate abscess formation. Perform bimanual examination by compressing the gland with one hand and by applying pressure in the direction of the respective salivary gland duct using the other hand. Assess for purulent discharge from the duct opening into the oral cavity. Also inspect the teeth, as dental abscess is one of the differential diagnoses. Laboratory tests usually reveal leukocytosis with predominance of neutrophils, and some advocate obtaining cultures of purulent drainage if present. Initial management includes appropriate antibiotics, hydration, sialogogues (such as lemon wedges), bimanual massage working in the direction of the duct opening in the oral cavity, warm compresses, appropriate pain control, and good oral hygiene. If there is no improvement in 2 to 3 days, or if abscess is suspected by physical examination, obtain a CT of the neck with contrast to assess for the presence of an abscess. If an abscess is present, surgical drainage is indicated. Once symptoms resolve, continue antibiotics for an additional week.[14]

Chronic sialadenitis usually results from sialolithiasis or salivary duct stenosis or compression. Obstruction results in salivary gland hypertrophy and fibrosis from chronic inflammation, and may lead to chronic pain of the involved gland. Patients usually report an initial episode of acute sialadenitis followed by repeated episodes of local pain and swelling. The underlying cause is often sialolithiasis, but may also include entities such as stricture of the salivary duct or compression from tumor. Physical examination is similar to acute sialadenitis, but finding the underlying cause is important. Evaluation may involve CT of the neck with contrast, among other studies. Management involves appropriately treating any episodes of acute sialadenitis (see previous section) and identifying and treating the underlying cause of the chronic inflammation.[14,15] In many cases, surgical excision of the involved gland is the definitive treatment.

Cervical lymphadenopathy may result from a variety of viral infections, including systemic infections such as human immunodeficiency virus (HIV), infectious mononucleosis (EBV), cytomegalovirus, or toxoplasmosis. Such infections may lead to cervical lymphadenopathy as well as more generalized lymph node involvement. A thorough history and review of systems is important to recognize the other symptoms of these systemic infections. On physical examination, it is important to note the location of the lymphadenopathy, size of the lymph nodes, mobility, lymph node consistency with respect to firmness, softness, or fluctuance, and tenderness to palpation. Diagnostic approach and treatment are determined by the suspected viral infection. After appropriate treatment, however, if the lymphadenopathy persists or enlarges, FNAB or referral to an otolaryngologist for possible lymph node biopsy is appropriate.[16]

Cat scratch disease is a bacterial infection caused by *Bartonella henselae*, which is transmitted by a cat scratch/bite or flea bite and often results in cervical lymphadenopathy. In the United States it generally occurs in young patients less than 21 years who are immunocompetent. History reveals exposure to kittens or to cats with flea infestation. Patients demonstrate regional, usually single node lymphadenopathy, and the location depends on the site of inoculation. The cervical region is one of the most common sites of involvement. The nodes are usually tender, possess overlying erythema of the skin, and are occasionally suppurative. Most involved nodes range in size from 1 to 5 cm. Patients also usually have a cutaneous lesion at the site of inoculation. Systemic involvement may occur, but less commonly than the cervical lymphadenopathy. Diagnosis is from history/physical examination and positive serology for *B henselae*. Treatment is medical using oral antibiotics.[17,18]

Tuberculous lymphadenitis in the cervical region, also known as scrofula, is a manifestation of extrapulmonary tuberculosis (*Mycobacterium tuberculosis*). Cervical lymphadenopathy is the most common manifestation of tuberculosis in the head and neck region. Patients most commonly present with multiple, matted, rubbery bilateral lymph nodes in the posterior cervical chain. Physical examination demonstrates firm, fixed masses in the posterior cervical region with or without overlying skin induration, a draining sinus, or fluctuance. Diagnosis is by FNAB, or occasionally excisional lymph node biopsy, following a positive PPD skin test, and other necessary tests to rule out pulmonary disease. A chest imaging study is always warranted when tuberculosis is suspected. Treatment usually involves a combination of 4 antitubercular medications. Complete excision becomes necessary when there is an actively draining sinus or fluctuance.[19]

Atypical or nontuberculous mycobacterial infections are usually seen in children and in immunocompromised patients (eg, HIV positive). These infections present as isolated disease, such as submandibular and submental cervical lymph node involvement. Patients rarely have constitutional symptoms. The atypical mycobacterial organisms are known to be resistant to antitubercular multidrug therapy. Due to this resistance, atypical mycobacterial infections are primarily treated with excision of the involved lymph node. Sometimes curettage is preferred to surgical excision. However, surgical management may not be necessary in all cases if the organism is sensitive to other antibiotics. However, surgical treatment is usually indicated in this type of infection.[20]

T: Trauma

Neck masses caused by trauma have a history and physical examination consistent with the type of trauma. A recent hematoma may reveal ecchymosis overlying a neck swelling, and is often tender to palpation and soft. In contrast, if the hematoma is well organized, it may become firm due to fibrosis. History and examination are diagnostic, and small hematomas usually resolve gradually without intervention. However, acute, expanding hematomas require surgical exploration and referral to an emergency department for immediate care.

Pseudoaneurysm or arteriovenous fistula may occur after shearing or penetrating trauma to the neck. Such a fistula may go unrecognized and later present as a soft, pulsatile mass with a thrill or bruit. A contrast-enhanced CT scan may assist in diagnosis, and treatment is surgical ligation.

Laryngocele may be caused by repeated use of musical instruments such as a trumpet. Diagnosis is established by history, physical examination, CT scan with contrast, and laryngoscopy if indicated. The lesion may continue to grow causing intermittent globus sensation, and serve as a nidus for infection. Surgical excision is definitive management.[15]

T: Toxic

Thyroid toxicosis is a biochemical disease entity that results from exposure to excessive concentrations of thyroid hormones. This disease state is 10-times more likely to occur in women. Graves disease is responsible for this condition in 60% to 85% of patients. Toxic nodular goiter results in 10% to 30% of cases while toxic thyroid adenoma is responsible for 2% to 20% of cases.[6,21] Thyroid disease is discussed in the article by Matthew C. Miller elsewhere in this issue.

E: Endocrine

Thyroid pathology is the leading cause of anterior neck compartment masses. The thyroid nodule is extremely common, occurring in 4% to 7% of the adult population, and about 5% of such nodules harbor a malignancy. Both of these thyroid conditions are discussed in the article by Matthew C. Miller elsewhere in this issue.

Parathyroid cysts are a rare entity but are clinically significant lesions. The literature reports 15% to 57% of parathyroid cysts as functional, although 33% is more commonly referenced. These functional cysts contribute approximately 1% to the cases of hyperparathyroidism.[22] The most common clinical presentation includes complaints of dysphagia with a female preponderance and greater than one-third demonstrating a palpable neck mass in the anterior cervical triangle. Symptoms of hypercalcemia-related hyperparathyroidism occur in the one-third of patients who harbor a functional parathyroid cyst. Other cystic lesions that may similarly present include branchial cleft cysts, cystic papillary carcinoma, and thyroglossal duct cysts, although thyroglossal duct cysts are usually midline masses that move with deglutition. As this differential diagnosis comprises surgical conditions, referral to an otolaryngologist with a good contrast-enhanced CT scan provides an adequate initial workup.

Another rare endocrine disease entity is parathyroid carcinoma, which accounts for approximately 1% of parathyroid pathologies. There is an equal sex distribution, and patients typically present during the sixth decade of life. The common features on presentation are those of hyperparathyroidism including fatigue, weight loss, psychiatric symptoms such as memory loss, muscular weakness, kidney stones, bone disease, and abdominal complaints such as constipation. The patient may have a breathy voice if the recurrent laryngeal nerve is invaded and there may be a palpable, firm mass that may trigger the diagnosis of parathyroid carcinoma when coupled with symptoms of hyperparathyroidism.[23,24] These symptoms should elicit a serum calcium level, a serum intact parathyroid hormone assay and referral to both an otolaryngologist and an endocrinologist. Contrast-enhanced CT scan of the neck is also beneficial in delineating the extent of disease and whether clinically significant lymph nodes are present.

N: Neoplasms

Adults older than 40 years have a high likelihood of harboring a malignant neoplasm. Malignant neoplasms as they relate to the upper aerodigestive tract are discussed in the article by Crozier and Sumer elsewhere in this issue. Some of the other more common benign and malignant neck neoplastic lesions are discussed here, including salivary gland neoplasms, primary vascular neoplasms, neurogenic neoplasms, and lymphoma.

The majority, that is, approximately 80%, of salivary gland neoplasms arise in the parotid gland. Neoplasms of the parotid gland are benign themselves approximately 80% of the time as well, while 50% of submandibular gland neoplasms are benign. Historically, patient tobacco and alcohol use are not associated with an increased incidence of salivary gland neoplasm, although some studies suggest an association of tobacco use with the development of a Warthin tumor. A history of radiation may increase the risk of benign pleomorphic adenoma or mucoepidermoid carcinoma. Occupational exposure to wood or silica dust is also associated with salivary gland malignancy.[25] Patients typically present with an asymptomatic neck mass anterior to the ear, inferior to the ear lobe corresponding to the tail of the parotid gland, or in the submandibular triangle. Tenderness to palpation is unusual but may occur with associated infection. Examination of the face or scalp may reveal a skin cancer that has metastasized to an intraparotid lymph node(s). A firm mass or facial nerve paresis is a poor prognostic finding associated with malignancy. A contrast-enhanced CT scan of the neck is warranted as well as FNAB for definitive surgical treatment.

Other common benign neoplasms presenting in the neck involve tumors arising from elements of the parapharyngeal space. These neoplasms include salivary gland tumors, neurogenic tumors, and paragangliomas (carotid body tumors, glomus jugulare, glomus vagale). The patient may complain of dysphagia, dyspnea, symptoms of obstructive sleep apnea, symptoms of eustachian tube dysfunction, or other symptoms related to cranial neuropathies. These symptoms usually present with significant tumor size. In addition, symptoms of flushing, hypertension, and palpitations may occur in association with functional paragangliomas. The most common finding on physical examination is that of a painless neck mass or painless oropharyngeal mass. The neck mass may have a palpable thrill or audible bruit. Paragangliomas derived from the carotid body are mobile in an anteroposterior direction but not in a vertical direction.[26] Patients with these symptoms and clinical findings warrant a contrast-enhanced CT scan of the neck, preferably from the skull base through the clavicles, before referral to an otolaryngologist. In addition, patients with symptoms of a secreting paraganglioma should undergo a 24-hour urine collection for catecholamines and their metabolites.

Lipomas and especially liposarcomas are extremely rare lesions presenting above the clavicles, as they usually occur in extremities and the trunk. In general, patients present with a slowly enlarging, painless neck mass. A history of trauma to the area affected may also be elicited.[27] Physical examination reveals a subcutaneous, smooth-surfaced soft tissue mass. A contrast-enhanced CT scan of the neck is warranted to determine the extent of the process before complete surgical excision.

Lymphomas are a heterogeneous group of lymphoproliferative disorders and are generally classified as Hodgkin or non-Hodgkin lymphoma. Symptoms include odynophagia, globus sensation, otalgia, or hearing loss associated with otitis media and dysphagia. Classic constitutional symptoms include fever, night sweats, and weight loss. Lymphomas present most frequently with lymphadenopathy and frequently involve the head and neck region. In the head and neck region this disease most often presents as a painless nodal mass. The mass may become painful with rapid growth. Hodgkin disease rarely presents in extranodal sites in the head and neck area, whereas non-Hodgkin lymphoma often presents with extranodal manifestation in the Waldeyer ring, mainly the palatine tonsil and nasopharynx.[28] CT imaging studies of the head and neck, chest, abdomen, and pelvis assist in staging, in addition to planning the most appropriate site for biopsy to confirm the diagnosis. Open biopsy is frequently necessary to ensure an adequate specimen for appropriate cytogenetic studies.

S: Systemic Diseases

There are a few rare systemic disease conditions with manifestation of neck masses as part of the disease entity. Such disease entities include Sjögren syndrome, sarcoidosis, Kimura disease, and Castleman disease. In addition, manifestation of the HIV systemically occurs frequently in the neck, as discussed previously with respect to infectious and neoplastic processes.

Primary Sjögren syndrome is a chronic disorder characterized by the Sicca complex of xerophthalmia with secondary keratoconjunctivitis and xerostomia. This syndrome is caused by immune-mediated destruction of the exocrine glands of lacrimation and salivation. Secondary Sjögren syndrome refers to the Sicca complex in association with other connective tissue disorders such as rheumatoid arthritis or systemic lupus erythematosus. This disease occurs in 1% of the population, with onset between the ages of 40 and 60 years and with a 9:1 female predilection. Approximately 80% of patients complain of xerostomia-related complications such as dysphagia, change in taste, fissures of the tongue and lips, and increased dental caries. Ocular symptoms include dryness, burning, foreign body sensation, and itching. Sinonasal complaints also occur, and manifest as epistaxis in 50% and hyposmia in 40% of patients. Approximately one-third of patients develop persistent salivary gland enlargement.[29] These symptoms should prompt an autoimmune serologic workup and referral to an otolaryngologist for a salivary gland biopsy, which is the single best diagnostic test.

Sarcoidosis is a multisystem disorder of unknown cause. Otolaryngologic manifestations of sarcoidosis occur in 10% to 15% of patients.[30] The most common sites of head and neck involvement are the cervical lymphatics, parotid glands, and facial nerve. Cervical adenopathy is the most common of the aforementioned head and neck manifestations, and was present in 48% of patients in a series by Dash and Kimmelman.[31] Referral to an otolaryngologist for diagnostic confirmation by FNAB or open biopsy demonstration of noncaseating granulomas is warranted.

Kimura disease is a chronic inflammatory condition characterized by a triad of painless subcutaneous masses in the head or neck region, blood and tissue eosinophilia, and markedly elevated serum immunoglobulin E levels.[32] This condition is endemic to Asian countries, although reported in America and Europe in Asian descendents. These patients are typically male, with a 76% incidence of subcutaneous soft tissue and deep cervical masses in the head and neck region on physical examination. These lesions are nontender and poorly circumscribed, commonly involving the periauricular, epicranial, and orbital regions of the head, and frequently manifest in the submandibular triangle (43%).[33] Patients may complain of pruritus and are most frequently free of systemic symptoms. A contrast-enhanced CT scan is nonspecific, usually demonstrating homogeneous-appearing lymph nodes with slight enlargement of the major salivary glands. The differential diagnosis includes lymphoma, scrofula, and eosinophilic granulomas. If the workup for tuberculosis is negative, referral to an otolaryngologist for biopsy is appropriate.

Castleman disease is an uncommon nonneoplastic lymphoproliferative disorder that can present as a solitary cervical lesion. Although this disease entity involves benign lymph node hyperplasia and usually affects the mediastinum, the second most commonly involved site is the head and neck area. The disease may manifest in a localized unicentric pattern with a slow-growing lymph node or as a multicentric systemic disease with numerous constitutional symptoms. Presenting signs and symptoms are generally nonspecific and therefore, Castleman disease should be considered in the differential diagnosis of long-standing inflammatory or neoplastic cervical masses.[34] A contrast-enhanced CT scan of the neck is helpful in defining the extent of disease. In addition, enhancement of the lesion differentiates this from lymphoma, which does not typically enhance. The diagnosis of Castleman disease is often difficult and when considered in the differential diagnosis, surgical excision with pathologic review is required to establish this diagnosis.

SUMMARY

The differential diagnosis for a neck mass is extensive and is easily remembered by employing the mnemonic "KITTENS" (**Table 1**),[3] which is an acronym for **K**—congenital/developmental anomalies, **I**—infectious/inflammatory, **T**—trauma, **T**—toxic, **E**—endocrine, **N**—neoplasms, and **S**—systemic diseases. Depending on the patient's age, the focus of this differential changes. For patients younger than 40 years the initial considerations should include congenital anomalies or infectious/inflammatory causes. In addition, traumatic origin of neck mass formation is also more common in this age group. However, for patients 40 years and older, 80% of neck masses are associated with a neoplastic process. Additional causes to consider for the development of a neck mass are endocrine pathologies and, more rarely, systemic disease.

ACKNOWLEDGMENTS

The authors would like to acknowledge Dawn Rosenberg for her artistic talent and preparation of our figure depicting the anatomic neck boundaries and lymphatic drainage patterns.

REFERENCES

1. Cummings CW, Flint PW, Harker LA, et al. Overview of diagnostic imaging of the head and neck. In: Otolaryngology—head and neck surgery. 4th edition. Philadelphia. Elsevier Mosby; 2005. p. 25–92.
2. Goffart Y, Hamoir M, Deron P, et al. Management of neck masses in adults. B-ENT 2005;1:133–42.
3. Pasha R. Otolaryngology: head and neck surgery clinical reference guide. 2nd edition. San Diego: Plural Publishing, Inc; 2006. p. 79, 207.
4. Bailey BJ, Johnson JT. Diagnosis and treatment of thyroid and parathyroid disorders. In: Head & neck surgery—otolaryngology. 4th edition. Philadelphia: Lippincott Williams & Wilkins; 2006. p. 1630.
5. Lin S, Tseng FY, Hsu CJ, et al. Thyroglossal duct cyst: a comparison between children and adults. Am J Otolaryngol 2008;29(2):83–7.
6. Cummings CW, Flint PW, Harker LA, et al. Differential diagnosis of neck masses. In: Otolaryngology—head and neck surgery. 4th edition. Philadelphia: Elsevier Mosby; 2005. p. 2540–53.
7. Huang S, Liao CT, Chin SC, et al. Transoral approach for plunging ranula: 10-year experience. Laryngoscope 2010;120(1):53–7.
8. Bailey BJ, Johnson JT. Salivary gland imaging. In: Head & neck surgery—otolaryngology. 4th edition. Philadelphia: Lippincott Williams & Wilkins; 2006. p. 538.

9. McGuirt WF. The neck mass. Med Clin North Am 1999;83(1):220–34.
10. Ro E, Thomas R, Isaacson G. Giant dermoid cyst of the neck can mimic a cystic hygroma: using MRI to differentiate cystic neck lesions. Int J Pediatr Otorhinolaryngol 2007;71:653–8.
11. Vaishali B, Nambiar A, Indudharan R. Lymphangioma of the larynx. J Laryngol Otol 2007;121(4):e2.
12. Bailey BJ, Johnson JT. Infections of the deep spaces of the neck. In: Head & neck surgery—otolaryngology. 4th edition. Philadelphia: Lippincott Williams & Wilkins; 2006. p. 665.
13. Fattahi T, Lyu P, Van Sickels J. Management of acute suppurative parotitis. J Oral Maxillofac Surg 2002;60:446–8.
14. Cummings CW, Flint PW, Harker LA, et al. Inflammatory disorders of the salivary glands. In: Otolaryngology—head and neck surgery. 4th edition. Philadelphia: Elsevier Mosby; 2005. p. 1323–38.
15. Schwetschenau E, Kelley DJ. The adult neck mass. Am Fam Physician 2002; 66(5):831–8.
16. Fletcher RH. Evaluation of peripheral lymphadenopathy in adults. In: UpToDate. Available at: http://www.uptodateonline.com/online/content/topic.do?topicKey= whitecel/8494&selectedTitle=1%7E150&source=search_result. Accessed January 26, 2010.
17. Spach DH, Kaplan SL. Treatment of cat scratch disease. In: UpToDate. Available at: http://www.uptodateonline.com/online/content/topic.do?topicKey=oth_ bact/4699&selectedTitle=2%7E44&source=search_result. Accessed January 26, 2010.
18. Spach DH, Kaplan SL. Microbiology, epidemiology, clinical manifestations, and diagnosis of cat scratch disease. In: UpToDate. Available at: http:// www.uptodateonline.com/online/content/topic.do?topicKey=oth_bact/5634& selectedTitle=1%7E44&source=search_result. Accessed January 26, 2010.
19. Spelman D. Tuberculous lymphadenitis. In: UpToDate. Available at: http://www. uptodateonline.com/online/content/topic.do?topicKey=tubercul/10671& selectedTitle=1%7E10&source=search_result. Accessed January 26, 2010.
20. Munck K, Mandpe AH. Mycobacterial infections of the head and neck. Otolaryngol Clin North Am 2003;36:569–76.
21. Vice CH, Hobgood C. Evaluating masses in the neck. Emerg Med 2004;36(9):20–8.
22. Ujiki MB, Nayar R, Sturgeon C, et al. Parathyroid cyst: often mistaken for a thyroid cyst. World J Surg 2007;31:60–4.
23. Myers EN, Suen JY, Myers JN, et al. Tumors of the parathyroid glands. In: Cancer of the head and neck. 4th edition. Philadelphia: Saunders; 2003. p. 472.
24. Okamoto T, Iihara M, Obara T, et al. Parathyroid carcinoma: etiology, diagnosis, and treatment. World J Surg 2009;33:2343–54.
25. Bailey BJ, Johnson JT. Salivary gland neoplasms. In: Head and neck surgery—otolaryngology. 4th edition. Philadelphia: Lippincott Williams & Wilkins; 2006. p. 1515–21.
26. Cohen SM, Burkey BB, Netterville JL. Surgical management of parapharyngeal space masses. Head Neck 2005;27:669–75.
27. Batsakis JG, Regezi JA, Rice DH. The pathology of head and neck tumors: fibroadipose tissue and skeletal muscle, part 8. Head Neck Surg 1980;3:145–68.
28. Myers EN, Suen JY, Myers JN, et al. Lymphomas presenting in the head and neck: current issues in diagnosis and management. In: Cancer of the head and neck. 4th edition. Philadelphia: Saunders; 2003. p. 601–10.

29. Bailey BJ, Johnson JT. Degenerative, idiopathic, and connective tissue diseases. In: Head and neck surgery—otolaryngology. 4th edition. Philadelphia: Lippincott Williams & Wilkins; 2006. p. 169–96.
30. Schwartzbauer HR, Tami TA. Ear, nose, and throat manifestations of sarcoidosis. Otolaryngol Clin North Am 2003;36:673–84.
31. Dash GI, Kimmelman CP. Head and neck manifestations of sarcoidosis. Laryngoscope 1988;98(1):50–3.
32. Thomas J, Jayachandran NV, Chandrasekhara PKS, et al. Kimura's disease—an unusual cause of lymphadenopathy in children. Clin Rheumatol 2008;27:675–7.
33. Sun QF, Xu DZ, Pan SH, et al. Kimura disease: review of the literature. Intern Med J 2008;38:668–74.
34. Markou KD, Goudakos JK, Psillas G, et al. Castleman's disease of the neck: report of a case and review of the literature. B-ENT 2009;5:189–93.

Head and Neck Cancer

Emily Crozier, MD, Baran D. Sumer, MD*

KEYWORDS

- Head and neck cancers • Surgical excision
- Radiation therapy • Chemotherapy

Nearly 650,000 people per year worldwide are newly diagnosed with head and neck cancer (HNCA). In the United States there were over 39,000 new cases of HNCA reported in 2005 and over 13,000 deaths attributed to HNCA.[1] Malignancies of the upper aerodigestive tract are varied in terms of location, presentation, and pathology. Anatomically, they include cancers of the paranasal sinuses and nasal cavity, nasopharynx, oropharynx, oral cavity, hypopharynx, and larynx. Although a tremendous variety of malignant processes can present in this region of the body, over 90% of HNCAs are squamous cell carcinoma.[2] The remainder of this article refers only to HNCA that is squamous cell carcinoma and excludes malignancies of the paranasal sinuses, nasal cavity, and nasopharynx, which are distinct subsites.

Although the mortality from HNCA has remained relatively constant over the last several decades, nonsurgical organ preservation strategies have been able to achieve oncologic results comparable to traditional radical surgery, while preserving greater function and improving the quality of life for patients with HNCA. In the meantime, traditional radical open surgery has been supplanted with minimally invasive transoral surgery that has led to greater functional preservation and good oncologic outcomes. Also reconstructive techniques have improved, giving head and neck surgeons the ability to remove larger tumors and reconstruct key anatomic subsites important for swallowing and speech.

As with many cancers, early detection of HNCA is the key to successful therapy. Primary care providers are the first line of detection for these varied tumors, and astute recognition of concerning symptoms and physical examination findings can lead to timely and appropriate referrals to an otolaryngologist or other appropriate specialist. Diagnostic delay due to physician-related variables (as opposed to patient-related delay), is an independent risk factor for decreased survival in laryngeal cancer, equivalent to having advanced-stage cancer.[3] Therefore, it is essential for primary care providers to have a good understanding of common findings on the history and physical examination of patients with HNCA.

Department of Otolaryngology–Head and Neck Surgery, University of Texas Southwestern Medical Center at Dallas, 5323 Harry Hines Boulevard, Dallas, TX 75390-9035, USA
* Corresponding author.
E-mail address: Baran.Sumer@UTSouthwestern.edu

Med Clin N Am 94 (2010) 1031–1046
doi:10.1016/j.mcna.2010.05.014
0025-7125/10/$ – see front matter © 2010 Elsevier Inc. All rights reserved.

This article reviews the pertinent clinical anatomy, epidemiology, pathogenesis, presenting signs, symptoms, and physical examination findings of HNCA; and will present a brief overview of the diagnostic work-up and treatment of HNCA.

ANATOMY AND FUNCTION

During the examination of a patient with complaints related to the upper aerodigestive tract, it is important to be familiar with the anatomic subsites that can potentially contribute to the patient's symptoms. A thorough knowledge of the head and neck anatomy will guide the relevant questions during the history and physical examination. This is critical because the location of a tumor determines its presentation and prognosis, as well as treatment. The boundaries between anatomic subsites can be difficult to distinguish, but precision in diagnosis can ultimately affect treatment success.

HNCA can be divided into several subsites that include the oral cavity, oropharynx, hypopharynx, and larynx. Cancers of the nasopharynx and thyroid and salivary glands, in addition to tumors of the nasal cavity, represent distinct pathologic entities and are not discussed in detail.

The oral cavity (**Fig. 1**) includes the mouth and its contents, from the lips to the junction of the hard and soft palates. Its inferior extent is the division between the oral tongue (the anterior two-thirds) and base of tongue, marked by the circumvallate papillae. The anterior tonsillar pillars mark the posterior extent; the palatine tonsils are not part of the oral cavity. The oral cavity, therefore, includes the lips, oral tongue, floor of mouth, vestibule (space between the teeth and cheek), hard palate, and alveolar ridges.

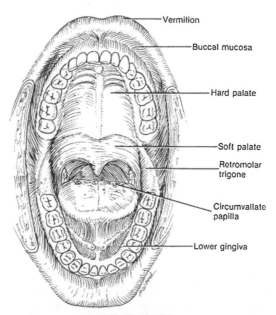

© 2005 Elsevier Science

Fig. 1. Overview of the oral cavity demonstrating the posterior boundary at the hard palate-soft palate junction and the location of the retromolar trigone relative to the inferior alveolar ridge. (*From* Wein RO, Malone JO, Weber RS. Malignant neoplasms of the oral cavity. In: Flint PW. Cummings otolaryngology: head & neck surgery, 5th edition. St Louis (MO): Mosby Elsevier; 2010; with permission.)

Immediately posterior to the oral cavity is the oropharynx. The tonsils and tonsillar pillars are part of the oropharynx and form the boundary with the oral cavity. The oropharynx includes the soft palate and uvula, tonsils, base of tongue (posterior one third of the tongue), and the pharyngeal walls (**Fig. 2**).

The hypopharynx is the continuation of the pharynx immediately inferior to the oropharynx (see **Fig. 2**). This region is difficult to visualize, but is composed of the space surrounding the larynx or the laryngopharynx. The hypopharynx is formed by the lateral and posterior pharyngeal walls and extends from the level of the hyoid superiorly to the esophageal inlet inferiorly. It includes the pyriform sinuses, two paired pyramidal recesses that flank the larynx and connect to the esophageal inlet. The postcricoid space immediately posterior to the larynx is also part of the hypopharynx.

Finally, the larynx can be divided into the supraglottis, the glottis, and the subglottis. The supraglottis includes the epiglottis, arytenoid cartilages, the aryepiglottic folds, and the false vocal cords. Just inferior is the true glottis, which consists of the true vocal cords and space 5 mm inferior to the level of the true vocal cords. The supraglottis and glottis are very distinct subsites of the larynx with different vascular and lymphatic supplies and patterns of tumor spread. The subglottis is the region of the larynx just inferior to the glottis, extending inferiorly to the cricoid cartilage.

The oral cavity, pharynx, and larynx interact in a complex way to control phonation, respiration, swallowing, and protection of the airway. Each of these functions is intricately associated with the other, and an alteration in one can affect the others. Airway protection is a priority during swallowing and, if not achieved, can lead to aspiration. The oral cavity functions in speech articulation, as well as the voluntary oral phase of

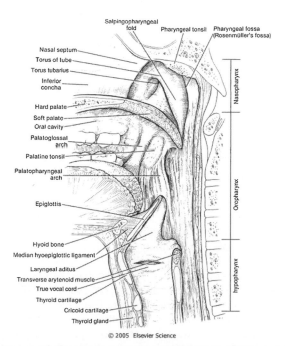

© 2005 Elsevier Science

Fig. 2. Surface anatomy of the oropharynx. (*From* Harreus U. Malignant neoplasms of the oropharynx. In: Flint PW. Cummings otolaryngology: head & neck surgery, 5th edition. St Louis (MO): Mosby Elsevier; 2010; with permission.)

swallowing, including mastication and preparation of the food bolus, and delivery of the bolus into the oropharynx. Once posterior to the tonsillar pillars, the involuntary oropharyngeal phase of swallowing commences. Alteration in these functions can be seen with oral cavity cancers.

During the involuntary pharyngeal phase of swallowing, the pharynx must contract sequentially to propel the food bolus into the esophageal inlet. The base of tongue contracts, pushing the food bolus posteriorly. Simultaneously, the soft palate is elevated against the posterior pharynx closing off the naso-pharynx. As the bolus is propelled posteriorly and inferiorly, the pharyngeal constrictors contract sequentially pushing the bolus inferiorly. Simultaneous contraction of the base of tongue, and elevation and anterior displacement of the larynx due to contractions of the strap musculature, folds the epiglottis over the airway. The glottis also closes to prevent aspiration. The elevation and anterior displacement of the laryngeal framework, coupled with opening of the cricophar-yngeus muscle at the esophageal inlet, creates negative pressure that propels the bolus past the larynx into the esophagus. During phonation, sound is created by the vibrations of the true vocal cords but, as the air column is propagated through the pharynx and oral cavity, the sound is altered and articulation using the oral tongue is achieved, resulting in more recognizable speech. Knowledge of the anatomy and physiology of these subsites coupled with a careful history and physical examination can give important clues with respect to tumor location even in subsites that cannot be directly visualized.

EPIDEMIOLOGY AND PATHOGENESIS

Cancers of the oral cavity, pharynx, and larynx represent a small overall percentage of new cancer cases each year. The American Cancer Society esti-mates the number of new cancers of the oral cavity and pharynx in the United States in 2009 to be 35,720 and the number of new cases of laryngeal cancer to be 12,290.[4] Males outnumber females in the number of new cases, but the proportion has been changing over the past several decades with the incidence of HNCA increasing in women. Even so, greater than twice as many men than women are affected by squamous cell carcinomas of the head and neck. The esti-mated number of deaths in 2009 is 3,660 for larynx cancer and 7,600 for oral cavity and pharyngeal cancers. For oral cavity and pharynx cancers, 1-year survival remains high, at 83%, with poorer 5- and 10-year survival rates of 60% and 49%, respectively.[4] A recent analysis showed that overall for HNCA, there was little change in survival or stage at diagnosis.[5] Subsite analysis revealed small but significant improvements in survival for patients with HNCA involving the oral cavity, nasopharynx, and oropharynx; and a significant but small decline in the survival for patients diagnosed with laryngeal cancer.[5]

HNCAs have had a strong association with tobacco and alcohol use. Tobacco and alcohol use are not only independent risk factors for the development of HNCAs, but their concurrent use has a multiplicative, rather than additive, effect on the risk of developing laryngeal cancer.[6] The use of smokeless tobacco has also been linked to cases of oral cavity cancer. The incidence of HNCA also tends to increase with age. The development of HNCA has a strong correlation with exposure to carcinogens such as tobacco and alcohol. In India and Southeast Asia, betel nut is chewed, sometimes in combination with lime and cured tobacco, and is associated with oral cavity cancer. As the Southeast Asian population in the United States has grown, this risk factor for oral cavity cancer has also become more common. These carcinogens induce genetic changes, either inactivating tumor suppressor genes or activating proto-oncogenes. Squamous cell carcinoma of the head and neck has been associated with alterations in the expression of p16, p53, pRb, and cyclin D1; as well as other oncogenes.

Another important marker whose expression is up-regulated in HNCA is the epidermal growth factor receptor, which is expressed in greater than 90% of HNCA. The expression levels correlate with decreased survival.[7,8] Vascular endothelial growth factor and its receptor are also involved in tumorigenesis and angiogenesis in multiple types of cancer, including HNCA, and may correlate with tumor progression.[9]

HIGH-RISK HUMAN PAPILLOMAVIRUS-RELATED HNCA

The importance of correctly evaluating and minimizing the morbidity of therapy for HNCA has become even more relevant with this changing epidemiology of HNCA. As smoking has declined in the United States, there has been a decrease in the overall incidence of HNCA over the last 15 years. Simultaneously, however, there has been an increase in the incidence of oropharyngeal cancer both in the United States and Western Europe.[10,11] High-risk variants of human papillomavirus (HPV), especially HPV-16, have been implicated as the cause for a subset of HNCA, especially of the oropharynx.[12] This is most likely due to changing sexual practices in the United States and Western Europe.[13,14] As the incidence of smoking-related HNCA has declined and the incidence of HPV related HNCA has increased, the proportion of HNCA caused by HPV has also increased.[11,14] Furthermore, HPV-related tumors appear to have a better prognosis and clinical outcome with both surgical and nonsurgical therapy.[15-17] One study from Sweden reviewed 150 cases of tonsil cancer from 1970 to 2002. Patients with HPV-positive tonsil cancer had 81% disease specific survival when compared with HPV-negative patients with 36% disease specific survival. These results were significant; were independent of age, tumor stage, and gender; and were true for each decade studied.[18] Other research corroborates these findings and confirms that smoking increases the risk of death from tonsil cancer and that HPV positivity in nonsmoking patients is linked with much higher disease-specific survival.[19] Fakhry and colleagues[15] showed the response to chemoradiation was improved in HPV-positive tumors (84% vs 57%) Also, Rich and colleagues[17] recently presented data supporting improved oncologic outcomes for HPV-related advanced oropharyngeal HNCA treated surgically. They report disease specific survival at 5 years was 91.7% versus 66.5%, for HPV-related and -unrelated HNCA of the oropharynx, respectively. Another study found that HPV infection status had a greater affect on prognosis than nodal metastasis in tonsil cancers.[20] The viral oncoproteins E6 and E7 interfere with tumor-suppressor proteins p53 and pRb, altering the normal regulatory mechanisms to curb cell growth and leading to an upregulation of p16. A trial evaluating patients treated with radiation showed that tumors positive for p16(INK4A) had improved locoregional tumor control, disease-specific survival, and improved overall survival.[21]

Additional risk factors for the development of upper aerodigestive tract cancers include familial cancer syndromes such as Li-Fraumeni or Fanconi anemia. A link between hypopharyngeal cancer and the iron-deficiency anemia associated with Plummer-Vinson syndrome has also been proposed.[22] Gastroesophageal reflux disease also has also been implicated as a potential contributing factor for laryngeal and pharyngeal cancer.[23-26]

PRESENTING SIGNS AND SYMPTOMS

Primary care providers are most often the first physicians to encounter patients with complaints related to the upper aerodigestive tract, including patients with neoplasms of this region. Careful history and examination can lead to prompt diagnosis and referral to an otolaryngologist or other appropriate specialist. There are some key symptoms and complaints that should not be ignored and, in certain patient populations, should raise concern for HNCA. In general, if a patient presents with a complaint related to the upper aerodigestive tract that does not resolve after initial treatment or intervention, this should raise concern for malignancy.

Knowledge of the anatomy of each subsite, as previously described, can guide history taking. Malignancies of the oral cavity often present as lesions of the tongue, gingivobuccal sulcus, buccal mucosa, or floor of mouth. Patients may complain of a nonhealing ulcer, area of irritation from adjacent teeth, pain, or bleeding. If present in the same location on repeat office visits, this should raise concern for malignancy. Although many entities in the oral cavity can mimic malignancy, any suspicious lesions should be biopsied for definitive diagnosis.

Nerve invasion, especially of the inferior alveolar nerve and the lingual nerve, can cause oral cavity or facial paresthesias. Patients may complain of tongue, lip, or chin numbness, although nerve invasion is usually a late sign for malignancies of the oral cavity. Lesions affecting the alveolar ridges can cause loose teeth, malocclusion, or poorly fitting dentures. Any of these symptoms in the presence of an oral lesion should raise concern. Lesions of the oral tongue or floor of mouth may cause dysarthria secondary to pain or mechanical fixation. Lesions affecting the tongue may also cause difficulty eating and manipulating a food bolus. Again, fixation of the tongue and interference with its mobility is a relatively late sign. If these symptoms are encountered in patients with a history of tobacco or alcohol use, malignancy should be high on the differential diagnosis.

Malignancies of the oropharynx often have more insidious symptoms. Patients may present with odynophagia or complain of otalgia. If physical examination of the ears does not reveal an obvious source for otalgia, it can represent referred pain from lesions of the pharynx due to cross-innervation by cranial nerves IX and X. Patients with HNCA of the pharynx and supraglottis can also present with a neck mass. Large neck masses that represent metastatic lymphadenopathy often originate from cancers in the pharynx or supraglottis that may themselves be too small to give other symptoms and may be difficult to detect with physical examination. Therefore, a neck mass, even with a normal examination of the upper aerodigestive tract, should still raise concern for malignancy. A neck mass in an adult patient is a malignancy until proven otherwise. Finally, oropharyngeal cancers can present with weight loss, because of odynophagia, but also because of the metabolic effects of the tumor.

Hypopharyngeal cancers can also be asymptomatic until they are quite advanced. Because of the proximity to the esophageal inlet, patients may complain of odynophagia or globus sensation. Often progressive dysphagia does not develop until the mass is quite large. As with the rest of the pharynx, patients with hypopharyngeal cancers may present with significant weight loss due to swallowing difficulty. These tumors can often invade the larynx and result in hoarseness or vocal cord paralysis, although this is also a relatively late sign.

HNCA of the glottis may be the easiest subsite to diagnose at an early stage. Patients will have significant and persistent hoarseness even with very small tumors only a few millimeters in size. If allowed to progress, this may develop into vocal cord paralysis with associated compromised aspiration or airway, both late findings in glottic cancers. Cancers of the glottis typically do not cause swallowing difficulty until they are very advanced. Supraglottic cancers, in contrast, do not cause hoarseness in their early stages, and may only cause odynophagia or referred otalgia. Finally supraglottic cancers can metastasize to regional lymph nodes quite early, which may be the only presenting sign; whereas glottis cancers typically do not metastasize until they are more advanced. Recognizing persistent symptoms and having a low threshold for referral is the key to early diagnosis.

PHYSICAL EXAMINATION

Patients presenting to a primary care physician with complaints related to the upper aerodigestive tract should undergo a full head and neck examination, including thorough examination of the ears, nose, oral cavity, and neck. Otoscopic examination should be performed to assess for the presence of middle ear fluid or other ear pathology. As patients with head and neck malignancies often present with otalgia, a primary ear pathology should be ruled out. Additionally, malignancies of the nasopharynx can obstruct the eustachian tube, creating negative middle ear pressure and serous effusions. Unilateral serous otitis media in an adult should raise concern for nasopharyngeal malignancy interfering with eustachian tube function. A patient complaining of otalgia in the absence of any clinical ear abnormalities should alert one to possible underlying malignancy.

The nasal cavity should be evaluated using a strong light to look for signs of epistaxis or nasal obstruction. Patients may complain of unilateral epistaxis or unilateral nasal obstruction with a large tumor of the paranasal sinuses or nasopharynx. Blood along the anterior nasal floor or anterior septum are more frequently due to trauma or dry air. Nasal obstruction may commonly be due to nasal polyps, rhinitis, a deviated nasal septum, or hypertrophied inferior turbinates. In the absence of these findings, patients with persistent unilateral nasal symptoms should be referred to an otolaryngologist.

The oral cavity examination should be performed with careful attention to the floor of mouth, the entire tongue surface, and the buccal mucosa. If the patient wears dentures, these should be removed before examining the oral cavity. A piece of gauze may be used to grasp the tongue and assist with visualization of the lateral edges and dorsal surface of the tongue. Oral cavity lesions should be palpated; firmness may indicate an underlying mass and immobility may indicate invasion into underlying tissues. One should perform a digital oral examination, palpating the floor of the mouth under the tongue and the tongue itself to feel for any firm masses. One should be aware of the presence of precancerous lesions such as leukoplakia and erythroplakia, which may present as white hyperkeratotic plaques that do not scrape off or erythematous plaques, respectively. These are considered clinical rather than pathologic diagnoses and may contain a range of abnormal cells from mild dysplasia to carcinoma-in-situ. Patients with leukoplakia have an increased incidence of oral cavity cancer and should be followed closely by an otolaryngologist, oral surgeon, or oral medicine specialist. The malignant transformation rates of oral leukoplakia have been shown to range from 17% to 24% in patients followed for more than 7 years.[27,28] Cancers of the oral cavity may also develop into erosive masses with destruction of teeth, the alveolar ridges, and even the mandible. Lichen planus that has the appearance of lacy white striae has also been associated with the development of oral cavity cancer.[29]

Examination of the oropharynx can be performed during the examination of the oral cavity. Careful attention should be paid to the tonsils, their symmetry, and the presence of any masses. Often, subtle irregularities in the contour or mucosal surface of the tonsil can signal a malignancy. Tonsil cancers can present as ulcerative lesions or exophytic masses. One should note the symmetry and motion of the soft palate and be alert for soft palate lesions. A tonsil cancer should not be confused with pharyngitis. A unilateral mass, ulcer, or plaque is concerning for malignancy; whereas pharyngitis may present with a generalized erythema or exudate.

Examination of the hypopharynx and larynx is much more difficult, as it requires either indirect mirror laryngoscopy or flexible fiberoptic laryngoscopy. A mirror examination can give a very good view of the base of tongue, supraglottis, and larynx; as well as the hypopharynx. Patients with a strong gag-reflex may be easier to examine with topical anesthesia usually provided with topical lidocaine. Patients with a large tongue or other anatomic variations that make it difficult to examine these areas require examination via flexible laryngoscopy by an otolaryngologist. Cancers of the larynx may present as mucosal irregularities, ulcerations, or exophytic masses. Objectively, however, the primary care provider may notice a hoarse, breathy voice or, in late-stage disease, stridor. Mucosal abnormalities, ulceration, bleeding, or pooled secretions in the pharynx or larynx should also raise suspicion and should be evaluated by an otolaryngologist.

Cancers of the oropharynx, hypopharynx, and supraglottic larynx may present initially with a neck mass. Most metastatic disease from these subsites present along the jugular chain of lymph nodes. Masses may be solitary or multiple and may have a cystic appearance on radiographic imaging. Lymph nodes involved with metastatic disease may not become fixed or firm until they are quite large; therefore, any appreciable neck mass in an adult should be evaluated with radiographic imaging using a CT scan or MRI and a fine-needle biopsy.

WORKUP

Suspicious head and neck lesions should be referred to an otolaryngologist. The otolaryngology examination will include a fiberoptic laryngoscopy, allowing excellent visualization of the entire upper aerodigestive tract, including the larynx and hypopharynx. With good topical anesthesia, flexible esophagoscopy, and bronchoscopy can also be performed in the office setting. There is up to a 10% incidence of second primary tumors in the upper aerodigestive tract in patients with HNCA, so careful examination may reveal an additional lesion.

Any concerning lesions identified on physical examination should be biopsied to obtain a tissue diagnosis. These biopsies can often be performed in the office setting with local anesthesia but may require a trip to the operating room for laryngoscopy with biopsy to obtain biopsies of difficult sites such as the base of tongue and to allow a thorough examination under anesthesia. Often, the concerning primary site is obvious and amenable to in-office biopsy. However, if the primary site of cancer is not known, an examination under anesthesia and biopsies of the nasopharynx, base of tongue, hypopharynx, pyriform sinuses, and tonsils will often reveal the source of nodal metastasis in patients where cervical lymphadenopathy is the only finding. The most common primary site for isolated nodal metastasis from HNCA is the oropharynx and nasopharynx.

A fine-needle aspiration (FNA) biopsy of the neck mass should be considered. Generally, this will be performed after appropriate imaging has been performed and is frequently done under ultrasound guidance. This allows the ultrasonographer to place the needle more accurately into the suspicious lesion, evaluate the lymph node for suspicious features such as central necrosis, and avoid inadvertently biopsying vascular lesions such as benign paragangliomas of the head and neck. These latter lesions should be easily distinguished from metastatic lymphadenopathy on imaging. The sensitivity, specificity, and accuracy of ultrasound-guided FNA for cervical lymph node metastasis has been estimated to be 89.6%, 96.5%, and 93.1%, respectively.[30,31] The main advantage of FNA is the avoidance of a surgical biopsy that can lead to scarring, potential tumor seeding, increased hospital stay, and increased costs. Furthermore, open surgical biopsy, if not well planned with respect to incision positioning, may interfere with definitive surgical management of HNCA.

In addition to tissue diagnosis, the initial workup should also include imaging studies. Imaging studies may be used to evaluate nodal involvement and to further evaluate findings on physical examination. CT scan with contrast is helpful for assessing cortical bone involvement, nodal status, including retropharyngeal nodes difficult to detect by other means, and involvement of adjacent structures such as the carotid artery or skull base. MRI may be indicated in some cases, especially for nasopharyngeal, parotid, or skull base tumors. In addition to obtaining CT scans of the neck, it is often necessary to obtain a CT scan of the chest to evaluate for metastatic disease or second primary tumors.

The use of positron emission tomography (PET) in conjunction with CT scanning, known as PET-CT, is useful in the evaluation of HNCAs. PET scanning relies on differential levels of radiolabeled glucose uptake in various tissues, with metabolically active tumors, including HNCA, showing increased uptake. PET-CT in HNCA is approved for evaluation for metastatic disease as well as for restaging after therapy is complete. It can be used to assess local and distant recurrence. Although it is sometimes used for identifying tumors of unknown primary origin (when lymphadenopathy is present with no known primary lesions) a careful panendoscopy with directed biopsies has great success in identifying primary tumors smaller than the effective resolution of PET-CT.[32]

Once this workup is completed, these cases should be presented at a multidisciplinary tumor conference with specialists from all treating fields to assess the case and formulate the appropriate treatment plans. These teams often include the head and neck surgeon, medical and radiation oncologists, radiologists, pathologists, and reconstructive surgeons.

COMMON PITFALLS

Several worrisome signs and symptoms should not be ignored in adult patients. Otalgia, especially if unilateral, should never be overlooked in an adult. It is quite unusual for an adult to develop otitis media, and this symptoms should be treated differently in an adult than in a child. Otitis externa will be evident on physical examination with tragal cartilage and canal tenderness; possible erythema; and edema and drainage from the ear canal. Referred otalgia can result from oral cavity, nasopharyngeal, oropharyngeal, and hypopharyngeal tumors; and should prompt a referral to an otolaryngologist.

A neck mass in an adult is cancer until proven otherwise. In the pediatric population, there are a variety of benign neck masses including thyroglossal duct cysts, branchial cleft cysts, reactive lymphadenopathy, and neck infections. All of these conditions are much less common in the adult population, and malignant lymphadenopathy must be highest on the differential. Cystic necrotic nodes may have a thin capsule surrounding a necrotic center that often mimics the appearance of a branchial cleft cyst on CT scan or MRI of the neck. One pitfall is to treat a neck mass with repeated courses of antibiotics, assuming that it is an infectious lymph node, without seeing improvement in the mass. A neck mass in an adult should trigger an immediate investigation, including CT scan with IV contrast, FNA, and referral to an otolaryngologist or head and neck surgeon.

Another common worrisome symptom is persistent hoarseness. Adults may experience laryngitis concurrently with an upper respiratory infection, or due to allergies or gastroesophageal reflux. But hoarseness that does not resolve after 3 to 4 weeks should not be ignored or treated with antibiotics. Persistent hoarseness is one of the most common symptoms of early glottic cancer and, because it is easily noticed, can lead to early diagnosis of larynx cancer if it is evaluated quickly.

Persistent sore throat should also raise concern. A typical viral pharyngitis may take 1 to 2 weeks to resolve but infectious causes such as tonsillitis or pharyngitis are much more common in children than adults. Sore throat that does not resolve in an adult, especially with no previous history of recurrent pharyngitis, should raise the possibility of HNCA. Localized or unilateral odynophagia should also raise concerns for malignancy. In fact, a general principle is that unilateral symptoms are much more concerning than bilateral complaints. Typically, infectious causes have a diffuse effect that does not result in unilateral pain or swelling. Finally, any persistent head and neck symptom that does not resolve with initial treatment may represent undetected HNCA rather than a treatment failure. If a patient has concerning symptoms that do not resolve with initial treatment, they should be referred to an otolaryngologist.

TREATMENT

All HNCAs are initially staged according to the tumor-node-metastasis staging system, which varies slightly by subsite, with assignments made based on tumor size and anatomic extent, nodal involvement, and the presence of distant metastases.[33]

The three most commonly used modalities to treat HNCA are surgical excision, radiation therapy, and chemotherapy. The anatomic location of the tumor, stage, size, involvement of adjacent normal structures, and the expertise available, all determine which modality or combination of treatments is recommended. Head and neck tumors can have complicated effects on patient quality of life and function with respect to speech and swallowing. Many of the structures affected by head and neck tumors are essential for mastication, swallowing, breathing, and communicating. Also, the head and neck is the most visible and noticeable portion of the human body, critical for social interactions and self-image. Treatments aim not only to cure the underlying malignancy, but to do so with as little functional and cosmetic morbidity as possible.

Recently, many trials have shown that chemotherapy with radiation is a viable treatment alternative to surgical excision for many subsites of HNCA.[34–39] The Veterans Affairs Laryngeal Cancer study showed induction chemotherapy followed by radiation resulted in equivalent survival and good organ preservation compared with radical open surgery followed by radiotherapy for advanced laryngeal cancer. The EORTC pyriform sinus cancer trial showed similar results for the hypopharynx subsite. RTOG 91-11 demonstrated improved local control for patients receiving concurrent chemoradiotherapy, compared with radiation alone, and induction chemotherapy followed by radiation. A meta-analysis by Pignon and colleagues[39] demonstrated a small but significant survival benefit to concurrent chemotherapy compared with adjuvant and neoadjuvant chemotherapy alone. Other trials have shown significant benefit to concurrent chemoradiotherapy compared with radiation alone for oropharyngeal cancers.[34,40–43] Based on these results, chemotherapy combined with radiation has also become a standard treatment for cancers of the oropharynx, which has improved rates of organ preservation and functional outcomes for patients with HNCA compared with traditional open surgical approaches to therapy. By undergoing nonsurgical treatment for their disease, patients with HNCA can potentially avoid radical surgery with its concomitant functional morbidity.

As nonsurgical therapy has evolved, however, primary surgical therapy also has improved over the last several decades. Chemotherapy has been added to radiotherapy in the postoperative setting and has been shown to improve locoregional control and improve progression-free survival for patients with advanced disease and adverse features such as extracapsular spread of cancer from regional lymph nodes.[44–47] Transoral surgical therapy has allowed improvements in functional preservation without compromising oncologic safety.[48] The evolution of surgery has culminated in transoral laser surgery as well as transoral robotic surgery, which can achieve good functional and oncologic outcomes for various subsites involved with HNCA, including the oropharynx.[48–57] This is true even for advanced-stage oropharyngeal tumors that in the past required open surgery with significant morbidity.[48,49,58] In one trial, patients with advanced base of tongue cancer treated with transoral laser surgery had excellent local control and survival, while most (73%) patients were able to tolerate a normal diet, with only 6% requiring permanent feeding tubes.[58] A recently presented study for Stage III and IV oropharyngeal cancer retrospectively followed 194 patients and reported overall survival at 2 and 5 years of 88% and 76.9%, respectively, with a long term gastrostomy dependence rate of 3.4%.[17] Also, reconstruction has improved with the greater use of microvascular techniques that allow free tissue transfer to replace excised tissue in the head and neck, improving functional outcomes for patients. There are a variety of tissue donor sites throughout the body that are accessible and have proved very versatile in head and neck reconstruction.

Both surgical and nonsurgical therapies represent continuously evolving and improving modalities for treating HNCA. In addition to organ preservation there is a shifting emphasis away from simple organ preservation to preservation of function. Typical postoperative doses of radiation are in the range of 56 to 66 Gy, while primary chemoradiotherapy delivers doses up to 74 Gy along with a radiosensitizing agent that increases the toxicity of the radiotherapy. Also, with primary surgery many patients that would have received chemotherapy with nonsurgical therapy can avoid chemotherapy altogether.[50] The question of which leads to greater morbidity remains unanswered: surgical resection or the extra dose of radiation with the addition of chemotherapy with nonsurgical therapy. There is compelling data to support both arguments but no currently prospective direct comparison.

Radiation therapy has also improved significantly over the past decades with more precision in terms of the radiated field. The use of intensity modulated radiotherapy allows radiation to be targeted to only the desired tumor and to avoid damage to surrounding tissues. It works by constantly reshaping the field and intensity of the beam based on the position of the tumor in relation to the moving treatment machine. It creates a differential between normal and cancerous tissue, with the goal of avoiding damage to healthy tissue. The result is fewer functional side effects and morbidity than the patient might have with standard radiotherapy or surgery. Proton beam therapy has also been investigated as a technique for minimizing the morbidity from radiation and minimizing the dose to critical structures such as the spinal cord.[59] Chemotherapy is used in conjunction with radiation for advanced HNCAs undergoing nonsurgical therapy and for the prevention of metastatic disease.[60,61] Epidermal growth factor receptor cetuximab has been shown to have biologic activity against HNCA and new targeted agents such as bevacizumab are currently in clinical trials.[62]

FOLLOW-UP

Patients with cancers of the head and neck have a unique set of challenges during their treatment, considering the critical functions the oral cavity, pharynx, and larynx perform. Maintaining adequate nutrition is a challenge in the setting of any cancer with its hypermetabolic effects. However, nutrition is especially problematic for patients with HNCAs because the cancer and its treatment often affect their ability to chew and swallow. Patients with larger tumors may present with severe nutritional deficiencies that must be addressed. Malnutrition may also have an adverse effect on the success of therapy. Poor nutrition can predispose patients to postoperative fistula and healing problems, and has been shown to be an independent negative prognostic sign with respect to oncologic outcomes for HNCA.[63] Surgical resections can permanently alter or temporarily impair the patient's ability to swallow, requiring nasogastric tube placement, or often gastrostomy tube placement for longer-term nutrition. Additionally, radiation therapy to the head and neck has enormous sequelae, with xerostomia resulting from salivary gland dysfunction and dysphagia resulting from pharyngeal fibrosis. Xerostomia may be treated with sialogogues, but the dysphagia may require feeding tube placement. Patients often need to be followed with serial laboratory studies to monitor nutritional status, and they need to have their weight carefully tracked during and after therapy. Additionally, larger tumors, as well as edema from radiotherapy, can lead to airway obstruction requiring a tracheostomy. Chronic aspiration due to the negative effects of therapy can also necessitate a tracheostomy. Physicians caring for these patients must be alert to sign of airway obstruction such as stridor. Suspected aspiration can be evaluated with a modified barium swallow study and evaluation by a speech pathologist who can assist patients in modifying their swallowing techniques to avoid aspiration. Patient with HNCA will often require speech therapy. Therapy for HNCA can affect speech and swallowing, requiring rehabilitation, and patients that undergo a total laryngectomy are unable to phonate normally at all because they lack a larynx. There are a variety of methods for rehabilitating speech for patients after a total laryngectomy, including the use of a electrolarynx, esophageal speech, and the use of a Blom-Singer speech prosthesis with a tracheo-esophageal puncture. Each of these modalities requires evaluation and training by a speech pathologist. Physical therapy also plays an important role in post-surgical rehabilitation.

One other longer term issue for HNCA patients may be tracheostomy care. Some patients require tracheostomy for airway protection before or during treatment. Tracheostomy placement alters the normal physiology of the airway, initially resulting in copious, thick secretions that require frequent suctioning. The use of humidified air via tracheostomy collar can help with clearance of secretions and compensate for the loss of normal humidification of air during inspiration by the nose. Important risk factors such as smoking and tobacco and alcohol use should be addressed, as second primary cancers and recurrence of the original tumor are not unusual.

SUMMARY

Cancers of the head and neck are complex in terms of presentation, anatomy, and treatment. Warning signs such as unilateral or persistent symptoms, otalgia, hoarseness, and neck masses should raise concerns for HNCA. The primary care physician plays a central role in this process of early diagnosis as many patients will initially present with symptoms to their primary physician. Timely diagnosis can improve functional and oncologic outcomes for these patients.

REFERENCES

1. Parkin DM, Bray F, Ferlay J, et al. Global cancer statistics, 2002. CA Cancer J Clin 2005;55(2):74–108.
2. Cohan DM, Popat S, Kaplan SE, et al. Oropharyngeal cancer: current understanding and management. Curr Opin Otolaryngol Head Neck Surg 2009; 17(2):88–94.
3. Teppo H, Koivunen P, Hyrynkangas K, et al. Diagnostic delays in laryngeal carcinoma: professional diagnostic delay is a strong independent predictor of survival. Head Neck 2003;25(5):389–94.
4. American Cancer Society. Cancer facts and figures. Available at: http://www.cancer.org/downloads/STT/500809web.pdf; 2009. Accessed December 30, 2009.
5. Cooper JS, Porter K, Mallin K, et al. National Cancer Database report on cancer of the head and neck: 10-year update. Head Neck 2009;31(6):748–58.
6. Talamini R, Bosetti C, La Vecchia C, et al. Combined effect of tobacco and alcohol on laryngeal cancer risk. a case-control study. Cancer Causes Control 2002;13(10):957–64.
7. Grandis JR, Tweardy DJ. Elevated levels of transforming growth factor alpha and epidermal growth factor receptor messenger RNA are early markers of carcinogenesis in head and neck cancer. Cancer Res 1993;53(15):3579–84.
8. Sok JC, Coppelli FM, Thomas SM, et al. Mutant epidermal growth factor receptor (EGFRvIII) contributes to head and neck cancer growth and resistance to EGFR targeting. Clin Cancer Res 2006;12(17):5064–73.
9. Mineta H, Miura K, Ogino T, et al. Prognostic value of vascular endothelial growth factor (VEGF) in head and neck squamous cell carcinomas. Br J Cancer 2000; 83(6):775–81.
10. Shiboski CH, Schmidt BL, Jordan RC. Tongue and tonsil carcinoma: increasing trends in the U.S. population ages 20–44 years. Cancer 2005;103(9):1843–9.
11. Vidal L, Gillison ML. Human papillomavirus in HNSCC: recognition of a distinct disease type. Hematol Oncol Clin North Am 2008;22(6):1125–42, vii.
12. Gillison MI, Koch WM, Capone RB, et al. Evidence for a causal association between human papillomavirus and a subset of head and neck cancers. J Natl Cancer Inst 2000;92(9):709–20.
13. D'Souza G, Kreimer AR, Viscidi R, et al. Case-control study of human papillomavirus and oropharyngeal cancer. N Engl J Med 2007;356(19):1944–56.
14. Chaturvedi AK, Engels EA, Anderson WF, et al. Incidence trends for human papillomavirus-related and -unrelated oral squamous cell carcinomas in the United States. J Clin Oncol 2008;26(4):612–9.
15. Fakhry C, Westra WH, Li S, et al. Improved survival of patients with human papillomavirus-positive head and neck squamous cell carcinoma in a prospective clinical trial. J Natl Cancer Inst 2008;100(4):261–9.
16. Weinberger PM, Yu Z, Haffty BG, et al. Molecular classification identifies a subset of human papillomavirus–associated oropharyngeal cancers with favorable prognosis. J Clin Oncol 2006;24(5):736–47.
17. Rich JT, Milov S, Lewis JS Jr, et al. Transoral laser microsurgery (TLM) +/- adjuvant therapy for advanced stage oropharyngeal cancer: outcomes and prognostic factors. Laryngoscope 2009;119(9):1709–19.

18. Lindquist D, Romanitan M, Hammarstedt L, et al. Human papillomavirus is a favourable prognostic factor in tonsillar cancer and its oncogenic role is supported by the expression of E6 and E7. Mol Oncol 2007;1(3):350–5.

19. Hafkamp HC, Manni JJ, Haesevoets A, et al. Marked differences in survival rate between smokers and nonsmokers with HPV 16-associated tonsillar carcinomas. Int J Cancer 2008;122(12):2656–64.

20. Straetmans JM, Olthof N, Mooren JJ, et al. Human papillomavirus reduces the prognostic value of nodal involvement in tonsillar squamous cell carcinomas. Laryngoscope 2009;119(10):1951–7.

21. Lassen P, Eriksen JG, Hamilton-Dutoit S, et al. Effect of HPV-associated p16INK4A expression on response to radiotherapy and survival in squamous cell carcinoma of the head and neck. J Clin Oncol 2009;27(12):1992–8.

22. Larsson LG, Sandstrom A, Westling P. Relationship of Plummer–Vinson disease to cancer of the upper alimentary tract in Sweden. Cancer Res 1975;35(11 Pt 2):3308–16.

23. El-Serag HB, Hepworth EJ, Lee P, et al. Gastroesophageal reflux disease is a risk factor for laryngeal and pharyngeal cancer. Am J Gastroenterol 2001;96(7):2013–8.

24. Vaezi MF, Qadeer MA, Lopez R, et al. Laryngeal cancer and gastroesophageal reflux disease: a case-control study. Am J Med 2006;119(9):768–76.

25. Qadeer MA, Colabianchi N, Strome M, et al. Gastroesophageal reflux and laryngeal cancer: causation or association? A critical review. Am J Otolaryngol 2006; 27(2):119–28.

26. Qadeer MA, Colabianchi N, Vaezi MF. Is GERD a risk factor for laryngeal cancer? Laryngoscope 2005;115(3):486–91.

27. Kawaguchi H, El-Naggar AK, Papadimitrakopoulou V, et al. Podoplanin: a novel marker for oral cancer risk in patients with oral premalignancy. J Clin Oncol 2008;26(3):354–60.

28. Silverman S Jr, Gorsky M, Lozada F. Oral leukoplakia and malignant transformation. A follow-up study of 257 patients. Cancer 1984;53(3):563–8.

29. Barnard NA, Scully C, Eveson JW, et al. Oral cancer development in patients with oral lichen planus. J Oral Pathol Med 1993;22(9):421–4.

30. Knappe M, Louw M, Gregor RT. Ultrasonography-guided fine-needle aspiration for the assessment of cervical metastases. Arch Otolaryngol Head Neck Surg 2000;126(9):1091–6.

31. Tandon S, Shahab R, Benton JI, et al. Fine-needle aspiration cytology in a regional head and neck cancer center: comparison with a systematic review and meta-analysis. Head Neck 2008;30(9):1246–52.

32. Lassen U, Daugaard G, Eigtved A, et al. 18F-FDG whole body positron emission tomography (PET) in patients with unknown primary tumours (UPT). Eur J Cancer 1999;35(7):1076–82.

33. National Cancer Institute. Available at: http://www.cancer.gov/. Accessed December 30, 2009.

34. Denis F, Garaud P, Bardet E, et al. Final results of the 94-01 French Head and Neck Oncology and Radiotherapy Group randomized trial comparing radiotherapy alone with concomitant radiochemotherapy in advanced-stage oropharynx carcinoma. J Clin Oncol 2004;22(1):69–76.

35. Induction chemotherapy plus radiation compared with surgery plus radiation in patients with advanced laryngeal cancer. The Department of Veterans Affairs Laryngeal Cancer Study Group. N Engl J Med 1991;324(24):1685–90.

36. Forastiere AA, Goepfert H, Maor M, et al. Concurrent chemotherapy and radiotherapy for organ preservation in advanced laryngeal cancer. N Engl J Med 2003;349(22):2091–8.

37. Lefebvre JL, Chevalier D, Luboinski B, et al. Larynx preservation in pyriform sinus cancer: preliminary results of a European Organization for Research and Treatment of Cancer phase III trial. EORTC Head and Neck Cancer Cooperative Group. J Natl Cancer Inst 1996;88(13):890–9.

38. Adelstein DJ, Saxton JP, Rybicki LA, et al. Multiagent concurrent chemoradiotherapy for locoregionally advanced squamous cell head and neck cancer: mature results from a single institution. J Clin Oncol 2006;24(7):1064–71.

39. Pignon JP, Bourhis J, Domenge C, et al. Chemotherapy added to locoregional treatment for head and neck squamous-cell carcinoma: three meta-analyses of updated individual data. MACH-NC Collaborative Group. Meta-analysis of chemotherapy on head and neck cancer. Lancet 2000;355(9208):949–55.

40. Adelstein DJ, Lavertu P, Saxton JP, et al. Mature results of a phase III randomized trial comparing concurrent chemoradiotherapy with radiation therapy alone in patients with stage III and IV squamous cell carcinoma of the head and neck. Cancer 2000;88(4):876–83.

41. Brizel DM, Albers ME, Fisher SR, et al. Hyperfractionated irradiation with or without concurrent chemotherapy for locally advanced head and neck cancer. N Engl J Med 1998;338(25):1798–804.

42. Calais G, Alfonsi M, Bardet E, et al. Randomized trial of radiation therapy versus concomitant chemotherapy and radiation therapy for advanced-stage oropharynx carcinoma. J Natl Cancer Inst 1999;91(24):2081–6.

43. Cmelak AJ, Li S, Goldwasser MA, et al. Phase II trial of chemoradiation for organ preservation in resectable stage III or IV squamous cell carcinomas of the larynx or oropharynx: results of Eastern Cooperative Oncology Group Study E2399. J Clin Oncol 2007;25(25):3971–7.

44. Cooper JS, Pajak TF, Forastiere AA, et al. Postoperative concurrent radiotherapy and chemotherapy for high-risk squamous-cell carcinoma of the head and neck. N Engl J Med 2004;350(19):1937–44.

45. Bernier J, Domenge C, Ozsahin M, et al. Postoperative irradiation with or without concomitant chemotherapy for locally advanced head and neck cancer. N Engl J Med 2004;350(19):1945–52.

46. Winquist E, Oliver T, Gilbert R. Postoperative chemoradiotherapy for advanced squamous cell carcinoma of the head and neck: a systematic review with meta-analysis. Head Neck 2007;29(1):38–46.

47. Bernier J, Cooper JS, Pajak TF, et al. Defining risk levels in locally advanced head and neck cancers: a comparative analysis of concurrent postoperative radiation plus chemotherapy trials of the EORTC (#22931) and RTOG (# 9501). Head Neck 2005;27(10):843–50.

48. Pradier O, Christiansen H, Schmidberger H, et al. Adjuvant radiotherapy after transoral laser microsurgery for advanced squamous carcinoma of the head and neck. Int J Radiat Oncol Biol Phys 2005;63(5):1368–77.

49. Jackel MC, Martin A, Steiner W. Twenty-five years experience with laser surgery for head and neck tumors: report of an international symposium, Gottingen, Germany, 2005. Eur Arch Otorhinolaryngol 2007;264(6):577–85.

50. O'Malley BW Jr, Weinstein GS, Snyder W, et al. Transoral robotic surgery (TORS) for base of tongue neoplasms. Laryngoscope 2006;116(8):1465–72.

51. Genden EM, Desai S, Sung CK. Transoral robotic surgery for the management of head and neck cancer: a preliminary experience. Head Neck 2009;31(3):283–9.

52. Park YM, Lee WJ, Lee JG, et al. Transoral robotic surgery (TORS) in laryngeal and hypopharyngeal cancer. J Laparoendosc Adv Surg Tech A 2009;19(3):361–8.

53. Hinni ML, Salassa JR, Grant DG, et al. Transoral laser microsurgery for advanced laryngeal cancer. Arch Otolaryngol Head Neck Surg 2007;133(12):1198–204.

54. Christiansen H, Hermann RM, Martin A, et al. Long-term follow-up after transoral laser microsurgery and adjuvant radiotherapy for advanced recurrent squamous cell carcinoma of the head and neck. Int J Radiat Oncol Biol Phys 2006;65(4): 1067–74.

55. Steiner W, Vogt P, Ambrosch P, et al. Transoral carbon dioxide laser microsurgery for recurrent glottic carcinoma after radiotherapy. Head Neck 2004;26(6):477–84.

56. Steiner W, Ambrosch P, Hess CF, et al. Organ preservation by transoral laser microsurgery in piriform sinus carcinoma. Otolaryngol Head Neck Surg 2001; 124(1):58–67.

57. Iro H, Waldfahrer F, Altendorf-Hofmann A, et al. Transoral laser surgery of supraglottic cancer: follow-up of 141 patients. Arch Otolaryngol Head Neck Surg 1998; 124(11):1245–50.

58. Steiner W, Fierek O, Ambrosch P, et al. Transoral laser microsurgery for squamous cell carcinoma of the base of the tongue. Arch Otolaryngol Head Neck Surg 2003;129(1):36–43.

59. Cozzi L, Fogliata A, Lomax A, et al. A treatment planning comparison of 3D conformal therapy, intensity modulated photon therapy and proton therapy for treatment of advanced head and neck tumours. Radiother Oncol 2001;61(3): 287–97.

60. Pignon JP, Baujat B, Bourhis J. [Individual patient data meta-analyses in head and neck carcinoma: what have we learnt?]. Cancer Radiother 2005;9(1):31–6 [in French].

61. Pignon JP, Bourhis J. Meta-analysis of chemotherapy in head and neck cancer: individual patient data vs literature data. Br J Cancer 1995;72(4):1062–3.

62. Bonner JA, Harari PM, Giralt J, et al. Radiotherapy plus cetuximab for squamous-cell carcinoma of the head and neck. N Engl J Med 2006;354(6):567–78.

63. Ravasco P, Monteiro-Grillo I, Marques Vidal P, et al. Impact of nutrition on outcome: a prospective randomized controlled trial in patients with head and neck cancer undergoing radiotherapy. Head Neck 2005;27(8):659–68.

Snoring and Obstructive Sleep Apnea

Seckin O. Ulualp, MD

KEYWORDS

- Snoring • Obstructive sleep apnea
- Sleep-disordered breathing • Positive airway pressure

Sleep is an essential aspect of the health and well-being of adults and children. Sleep disorders including, but not limited to, insomnia, narcolepsy, restless leg syndrome, and sleep apnea, lead to reduced quality of life and productivity as well as increased use of health care services.[1] It is estimated that 50 to 70 million individuals in United States are affected by sleep problems.[1] Symptoms of sleep disruption are reported in 30% of the general population.[2] In the primary care setting more than 50% of patients have sleep complaints.[2] Primary care physicians are critical in early recognition, treatment, and long-term management of individuals with sleep disorders. The complex nature of sleep-related medical and behavioral problems requires multidisciplinary assessment and management.

Otolaryngologists are commonly asked to evaluate adults and children with snoring and obstructive sleep apnea (OSA). Snoring is estimated to occur in 3% to 12% of children[3-5] and up to 59% of adults.[6,7] Snoring is associated with OSA. OSA is a reduction or complete cessation in breathing due to obstruction of the upper airway after the initiation of sleep, which disrupts normal ventilation and sleep patterns.[8,9] Patients with OSA present with a variety of symptoms including excessive daytime sleepiness, snoring, unrefreshing sleep, fatigue, insomnia, episodes of gasping for air, or choking. OSA may be associated with myriad clinical consequences such as increased risk of systemic hypertension, coronary vascular disease, congestive heart failure, cerebrovascular disease, glucose intolerance, impotence, obesity, pulmonary hypertension, gastroesophageal reflux, and impaired concentration.[1,10-16] OSA is estimated to occur in between 5% and 10% of the United States population.[17,18] The prevalence of high risk of OSA in the Unites States is 26%.[7] Despite the relatively high prevalence of OSA, diagnosis and treatment may be delayed. Nonetheless, OSA remains undiagnosed in 82% of men and 93% of women with the condition.[19] Early identification and treatment of OSA provides significant relief for individuals, prevents complications of OSA, and reduces overall health care costs.[20,21] Better understanding of the pathogenesis, risk factors, diagnosis and treatment of OSA has the potential to improve

Department of Otolaryngology-Head and Neck Surgery, University of Texas Southwestern Medical Center, 5323 Harry Hines Boulevard, Dallas, TX 75390-9035, USA
E-mail address: seckin.ulualp@utsouthwestern.edu

Med Clin N Am 94 (2010) 1047–1055
doi:10.1016/j.mcna.2010.05.002
0025-7125/10/$ – see front matter © 2010 Elsevier Inc. All rights reserved.

early recognition of OSA and prevention of adverse effects on the individual and society.

PATHOGENESIS

OSA is a common disorder resulting from collapse of the upper airway. Air flow is affected by size, compliance, and shape of the upper airway. The framework of the upper airway consists of bones including the nasal turbinates, maxilla, mandible, hyoid, cervical vertebrae, and soft tissues including the adenoid, soft palate, tonsillar pillars, tonsils, uvula, soft palate, pharyngeal fat pad and mucosa, pharyngeal muscles, and epiglottis. Upper airway patency is accomplished by complex interactions among anatomic structures, neuromuscular tone, ventilatory control mechanisms, level of consciousness, upper airway reflexes, peripheral nervous system mechanisms, body position, vascular tone, surface tension forces, lung volume effects, and expiratory collapse.[22]

Obstructive apnea or hypopnea occurs due to intermittent complete and partial obstruction of the nose and the pharynx. Nasal obstruction has been implicated in the pathogenesis of OSA by increasing airway resistance that predisposes pharyngeal collapse, reducing nasal afferent reflexes maintaining muscular tone, reducing humidification leading to increased surface tension, and increasing the tendency for breathing through the mouth, destabilizing the lower pharyngeal airway by displacing the hyoid.[23–26]

Soft tissues, skeletal morphology, and obesity influence the upper airway configuration. The pharyngeal lumen appears to be circular or elliptical, with the long axis in the anterior-posterior dimension due to medial displacement of the lateral pharyngeal walls in OSA.[27] Micrognathia and retrognathia are common structural abnormalities that cause displacement of the tongue, soft palate, and soft tissues, leading to impingement of the airway.[28,29] Inferior displacement of the hyoid bone with associated inferior displacement of the tongue into the hypopharyngeal area is suggested to reduce the size of the pharyngeal lumen in patients with OSA.[30,31] Larger volumes of the adenoid, tonsil, lateral pharyngeal wall, tongue, and soft palate, and thickening of the lateral pharyngeal walls are reported in OSA.[32–38] Obesity contributes to the pathogenesis of OSA by increasing the fat distribution around the neck and airway and by altering the metabolism and ventilation via leptin and other cytokines, which increase carbon dioxide response thus causing central ventilatory sensitivity.[39,40]

The airway size is changed with body positioning. Patients with OSA have a greater decrease in airway size following positioning from sitting to supine.[41] In addition to the change in size of the airway, airway collapsibility is altered in OSA. Patients with OSA are reported to have a more collapsible pharyngeal airway than control subjects.[42,43] The role of pharyngeal muscles such as the tensor veli palatini and genioglossus in maintaining a patent airway has been studied in normal individuals and in patients with OSA. The tensor palatini tenses the soft palate and the genioglossus protrudes and depresses the tongue. During apneic events, genioglossus activity increases in response to an increase in carbon dioxide pressure until the patient awakens.[44]

DIAGNOSIS

Early identification of OSA relies on a high level of suspicion of the primary care physician. A careful sleep history is a critical part of the evaluation of patients with OSA. During a routine health maintenance evaluation, screening for OSA can be performed by inquiring about snoring, daytime sleepiness, obesity, hypertension, or retrognathia.[45] More comprehensive sleep history and physical examination are necessary patients with positive findings in screening and patients at high risk for OSA. Presence of obesity (body mass index [BMI; weight in kilograms divided by height in meters squared] >35), congestive heart failure, atrial fibrillation, treatment of refractory hypertension, type 2 diabetes, nocturnal dysrhythmias, stroke, pulmonary hypertension, high-risk driving populations, or preparation for bariatric surgery indicates patients at high risk for OSA.[45]

Comprehensive sleep history includes evaluation of witnessed apneas, snoring, gasping/choking at night, excessive sleepiness, nonrefreshing sleep, total sleep amount, nocturia, morning headaches, decreased concentration, memory loss, decreased libido, irritability, sleep fragmentation/maintenance insomnia, and sleepiness severity as measured by the by Epworth Sleepiness Scale.[45] The degree of daytime sleepiness in OSA shows interindividual differences. In addition to OSA, coexisting conditions such as diabetes, chronic obstructive pulmonary disease, obesity hypoventilation syndrome, level of exercise, and emotional stress may influence the presence and degree of daytime sleepiness.[46,47] The association between excessive daytime sleepiness and severity of OSA has been reported, with varying results.[48–50] The Epworth Sleepiness Scale is used to determine the daytime sleepiness based on likelihood of dozing or sleeping during the following 8 everyday activities: sitting and reading, watching TV, sitting inactive in a public place, being a passenger in a motor vehicle for an hour or more, lying down in the afternoon, sitting and talking to someone, sitting quietly after lunch (no alcohol), and stopping for a few minutes in traffic (**Table 1**).[51] The chance of sleeping or dozing for each situation is graded using the following scale: 0 = would never doze or sleep, 1 = slight chance of dozing or sleeping, 2 = moderate chance of sleeping or dozing, 3 = high chance of dozing or sleeping (see **Table 1**).[51] The patient chooses the most appropriate number for each situation. A score of 10 or more is considered sleepy and a score of 16 or more is very sleepy.

Table 1
Items and scale of Epworth sleepiness scale

Situation	Chance of Dozing or Sleeping			
	0	1	2	3
Sitting and reading				
Watching TV				
Sitting, inactive in a public place				
As a passenger in a car for an hour without a break				
Lying down to rest in the afternoon when circumstances permit				
Sitting and talking to someone				
Sitting quietly after a lunch without alcohol				
In a car while stopped for a few minutes in the traffic				

0, would never doze; 1, slight chance of dozing; 2, moderate chance of dozing; 3, high chance of dozing.

Data from Johns MW. A new method for measuring daytime sleepiness: the Epworth sleepiness scale. Sleep 1991;14:540–5.

The physical examination should include respiratory, cardiovascular, and neurologic systems. The presence of increased neck circumference, BMI 30 or more, modified Mallampati score of 3 or 4 (**Fig. 1**),[52,53] retrognathia, lateral peritonsillar narrowing, macroglossia, tonsillar hypertrophy, elongated/enlarged uvula, high arched/narrow hard palate, or nasal abnormalities may suggest the presence of OSA.[45] Patients with suspected OSA should be evaluated for eligibility for surgery during general sleep evaluation.

Patients at high risk for OSA need to have objective testing to confirm the diagnosis and to determine the severity of the disease. Patients who are not at high risk for OSA may need objective testing depending on the risk of OSA, presence of daytime impairment, or other morbidities.[45] The diagnosis of OSA can be established using 2 acceptable methods: (1) polysomnography and (2) home testing with portable monitors. Polysomnography is routinely indicated for the diagnosis of sleep-related breathing disorders.[54] High-risk patients with nocturnal symptoms of OSA, and patients who are scheduled for upper airway surgery for snoring and OSA should undergo sleep testing.[54] Polysomnography is recommended to determine the presence of OSA in patients who are scheduled for bariatric surgery.[45] Home testing with portable monitors may be used to monitor response to positive airway pressure treatment and diagnose OSA in patients who cannot undergo in-laboratory polysomnography. Follow-up polysomnography or attendant cardiorespiratory monitoring (type 3 portable monitoring) is needed for postsurgical assessment of moderate to severe OSA and to ensure therapeutic benefit from an oral appliance.[54,55] Response to continuous positive airway pressure treatment should be monitored after substantial weight loss, such as 10% of body weight, substantial weight gain with return of symptoms, or insufficient clinical response.[54]

TREATMENT

The treatment of OSA includes medical, behavioral, and surgical options presented in a multidisciplinary setting. Following the review of results of the objective testing with the patient, the patient should be educated in the pathophysiology, risk factors, natural history, and clinical consequences of OSA.[45] Information on the role of weight

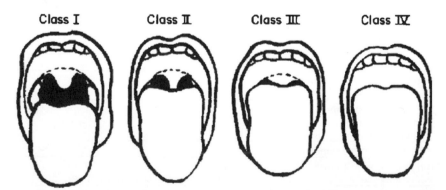

Fig. 1. Mallampati scores. (*Reprinted from* Bair AE, Caravelli R, Tyler K, et al. Feasibility of the preoperative Mallampati airway assessment in Emergency Department patients. J Emerg Med 2010;38[5]:677–80. DOI: 10.1016/j.jemermed.2008.12.019; with permission from Elsevier. *Data from* Kushida CA, Littner MR, Morgenthaler T, et al. Practice parameters for the indications for polysomnography and related procedures: an update for 2005. Sleep 2005;28:499–521.)

loss, risk factor modification, effects of medication, and behavioral approaches, such as avoiding alcohol and sedatives near bedtime and avoiding the supine position, have to be presented.[45] The patient should be counseled on the risks and management of drowsy driving.[45]

Positive airway pressure treatment should be offered as an option to all patients. Alternative therapies such as behavioral strategies, oral appliances, surgical options, and adjunctive therapies are offered depending on the severity of the OSA as well as presence of anatomic abnormalities and other risk factors. Before positive airway pressure treatment, the patient should be educated about the function, care, and maintenance of their equipment, benefits of treatment, and potential problems. The usage of positive airway pressure treatment should be monitored with time meters.[56]

Oral appliances may be used to improve upper airway patency during sleep by decreasing upper airway collapsibility.[57] Mandibular repositioning appliances and tongue-retaining devices have been used to hold the mandible in an advanced position and the tongue in a forward position. Oral appliances are used in patients with mild to moderate OSA who are not candidates for positive airway pressure treatment.[55] A dental examination consisting of dental history and complete intraoral examination should be performed to determine candidacy for oral appliances. A polysomnogram or an attendant cardiorespiratory sleep study should be obtained after final adjustment of the oral appliance.[55]

Surgical treatment of OSA includes a wide variety of procedures targeting relief of obstruction at different levels of the airway. During the initial general sleep evaluation the patients should be evaluated for anatomic abnormalities to identify possible surgical sites. After establishing the diagnosis of OSA, patients should be counseled on the surgical options, goals of treatment, success rate, risks and benefits of the procedure, complications, alternative treatments, and side effects.[45] Surgical procedure may be considered as a secondary treatment for inadequate treatment outcome from positive airway pressure treatment and oral appliances. Long-term follow-up with a sleep specialist is recommended after surgical treatment.[45]

Adjunctive therapies of OSA include bariatric surgery, pharmacologic agents, and oxygen therapy. Bariatric surgery can be considered as an adjunctive treatment for obese patients with OSA. Bariatric surgery is indicated in individuals with a BMI of 40 or more, or BMI of 35 or more with comorbidities.[58] Topical nasal steroids can be used in the presence of concurrent rhinitis.[59] Modafinil is recommended for treatment of residual excessive daytime sleepiness despite positive airway pressure treatment.[59]

SUMMARY

OSA is characterized by reduction or complete cessation in breathing due to obstruction of the upper airway after the initiation of sleep, which disrupts normal ventilation and sleep patterns.[8,9] Patients with OSA present with a variety of symptoms including excessive daytime sleepiness, snoring, unrefreshing sleep, fatigue, insomnia, episodes of gasping for air, or choking. OSA may be associated with clinical consequences such as increased risk of systemic hypertension, congestive heart failure, cerebrovascular disease, glucose intolerance, impotence, obesity, pulmonary hypertension, gastroesophageal reflux, and impaired concentration. Early identification and treatment of OSA provides significant relief for individuals, prevents complications of OSA, and reduces overall health care costs.[20,21]

A careful sleep history is a critical part of the evaluation of patients with OSA. During a routine health maintenance evaluation, screening for OSA can be performed by inquiring about snoring, daytime sleepiness, obesity, hypertension, or retrognathia. More comprehensive sleep history and physical examination are necessary for patients with positive findings in screening and patients at high risk for OSA. Presence of obesity (BMI >35), congestive heart failure, atrial fibrillation, treatment of refractory hypertension, type 2 diabetes, nocturnal dysrhythmias, stroke, pulmonary hypertension, high-risk driving populations, or preparation for bariatric surgery indicates patients at high risk for OSA.[45] Patients at high risk for OSA need to have objective testing to confirm the diagnosis and to determine the severity of the disease. Patients who are not at high risk for OSA may need objective testing depending on the risk of OSA, presence of daytime impairment, or other morbidities.[45] The treatment of OSA includes medical, behavioral, and surgical options presented in a multidisciplinary setting, and therapeutic approaches should be individualized to the severity of apnea and the patient's desire.

REFERENCES

1. Institute of Medicine. Sleep disorders and sleep deprivation: an unmet public health problem. Washington, DC: The National Academies Press; 2006. Available at: http://www.iom.edu/cms/3740/23160/33668.aspx. Accessed November 24, 2009.
2. Pagel JF. Obstructive sleep apnea (OSA) in primary care: evidence-based practice. J Am Board Fam Med 2007;20(4):392–8.
3. Ali NJ, Pitson D, Stradling JR. Natural history of snoring and related behaviour problems between the ages of 4 and 7 years. Arch Dis Child 1994;71(1): 74–6.
4. Gislason T, Benediktsdóttir B. Snoring, apneic episodes, and nocturnal hypoxemia among children 6 months to 6 years old. An epidemiologic study of lower limit of prevalence. Chest 1995;107(4):963–6.
5. Hultcrantz E, Löfstrand-Tideström B, Ahlquist-Rastad J. The epidemiology of sleep related breathing disorder in children. Int J Pediatr Otorhinolaryngol 1995;32(Suppl):S63–6.
6. Young T, Palta M, Dempsey J, et al. The occurrence of sleep-disordered breathing among middle-aged adults. N Engl J Med 1993;328:1230–5.
7. Hiestand DM, Britz P, Goldman M, et al. Prevalence of symptoms and risk of sleep apnea in the US population: results from the national sleep foundation sleep in America 2005 poll. Chest 2006;130(3):780–6.
8. American Toracic Society. Standards and indications for cardiopulmonary sleep studies in children. American Thoracic Society. Am J Respir Crit Care Med 1996;153(2):866–78.
9. Gatsaut H, Tassinari CA, Duron B. Polygraphic study of the episodic diurnal and nocturnal (hypnic and respiratory) manifestations of the Pickwick syndrome. Brain Res 1966;1:167–86.
10. Nieto FJ, Young TB, Lind BK, et al. Association of sleep-disordered breathing, sleep apnea, and hypertension in a large community-based study. JAMA 2000; 283:1829–36.
11. Peppard PE, Young T, Palta M, et al. Prospective study of the association between sleep-disordered breathing and hypertension. N Engl J Med 2000; 342:1378–84.
12. Peker Y, Hedner J, Norum J, et al. Increased incidence of cardiovascular disease in middle-aged men with obstructive sleep apnea: a 7-year follow-up. Am J Respir Crit Care Med 2002;166:159–65.

13. Kaneko Y, Floras JS, Usui K, et al. Cardiovascular effects of continuous positive airway pressure in patients with heart failure and obstructive sleep apnea. N Engl J Med 2003;348:1233–41.
14. Yaggi HK, Concat J, Kernan WN, et al. Obstructive sleep apnea as a risk factor for stroke and death. N Engl J Med 2005;343:2034–41.
15. Babu AR, Herdegen J, Fogelfeld L, et al. Type 2 diabetes, glycemic control, and continuous positive airway pressure in obstructive sleep apnea. Arch Intern Med 2005;165:447–52.
16. Goncalves MA, Guilleminault C, Ramos E, et al. Erectile dysfunction, obstructive sleep apnea syndrome, and nasal CPAP treatment. Sleep Med 2005;6: 333–9.
17. Tishler PV, Larkin EK, Schluchter MD, et al. Incidence of sleep-disordered breathing in an urban adult population: the relative importance of risk factors in the development of sleep-disordered breathing. JAMA 2003;289:2230–7.
18. Young T, Peppard PE, Gottlieb DJ. Epidemiology of obstructive sleep apnea: a population health perspective. Am J Respir Crit Care Med 2002;165:1217–39.
19. Young T, Evans L, Finn L, et al. Estimation of the clinically diagnosed proportion of sleep apnea syndrome in middle-aged men and women. Sleep 1997;20:705–6.
20. Kryger MH, Roos L, Delaive K, et al. Utilization of healthcare services in patients with severe obstructive sleep apnea. Sleep 1996;19(Suppl 9):S111–6, 4.
21. Peker Y, Hedner J, Johannsson A, et al. Reduced hospitalization with cardiovascular and pulmonary disease in obstructive sleep apnea patients on nasal CPAP treatment. Sleep 1997;20(8):645–53.
22. Woodson BT, Franco R. Physiology of sleep disordered breathing. Otolaryngol Clin North Am 2007;40(4):691–711.
23. Young T, Finn L, Kim H. Nasal obstruction as a risk factor for sleep-disordered breathing. The University of Wisconsin Sleep and Respiratory Research Group. J Allergy Clin Immunol 1997;99:757–62.
24. Meurice J, Marc I, Carrier G, et al. Effects of mouth opening on upper airway collapsibility in normal sleeping subjects. Am J Respir Crit Care Med 1996;153: 255–9.
25. Schwab RJ, Gefter WB, Hoffman EA, et al. Dynamic upper airway imaging during respiration in normal subjects and patients with sleep disordered breathing. Am Rev Respir Dis 1993;148:1385–400.
26. Schwab RJ, Pairstein M, Pierson R, et al. Identification of upper airway anatomic risk factors for obstructive sleep apnea with volumetric MRI. Am J Respir Crit Care Med 2003;167(9):1176–80.
27. Bradley TD, Brown IG, Grossman RF, et al. Pharyngeal size in snorers, nonsnorers, and patients with obstructive sleep apnea. N Engl J Med 1986;315(21): 1327–31.
28. Ferguson KA, Ono T, Lowe AA, et al. The relationship between obesity and craniofacial structure in obstructive sleep apnea. Chest 1995;108:375–81.
29. Watanabe T, Isono S, Tanaka A, et al. Contribution of body habitus and craniofacial characteristics to segmental closing pressures of the passive pharynx in patients with sleep-disordered breathing. Am J Respir Crit Care Med 2002;165: 260–5.
30. Young JW, McDonald JP. An investigation into the relationship between the severity of obstructive sleep apnoea/hypopnoea syndrome and the vertical position of the hyoid bone. Surgeon 2004;2:145–51.
31. Riha RL, Brander P, Vennelle M, et al. A cephalometric comparison of patients with sleep apnea/hypopnea syndrome and their siblings. Sleep 2005;28:315–20.

32. Schwab RJ, Pasirstein M, Pierson R, et al. Identification of upper airway anatomic risk factors for obstructive sleep apnea with volumetric magnetic resonance imaging. Am J Respir Crit Care Med 2003;168:522–30.

33. Schellenberg JB, Maislin G, Schwab RJ. Physical findings and the risk for obstructive sleep apnea. The importance of oropharyngeal structures. Am J Respir Crit Care Med 2000;162:740–8.

34. Schwab RJ, Gupta KB, Gefter WB, et al. Upper airway and soft tissue anatomy in normal subjects and patients with sleep-disordered breathing. Significance of the lateral pharyngeal walls. Am J Respir Crit Care Med 1995;152:1673–89.

35. Greenfeld M, Tauman R, DeRowe A, et al. Obstructive sleep apnea syndrome due to adenotonsillar hypertrophy in infants. Int J Pediatr Otorhinolaryngol 2003;67:1055–60.

36. Bradley TD, Rutherford R, Grossman RF, et al. Role of daytime hypoxemia in the pathogenesis of right heart failure in the obstructive sleep apnea syndrome. Am Rev Respir Dis 1985;131:835–9.

37. Ingman T, Nieminen T, Hurmerinta K. Cephalometric comparison of pharyngeal changes in subjects with upper airway resistance syndrome or obstructive sleep apnoea in upright and supine positions. Eur J Orthod 2004;26:321–6.

38. Stauffer JL, Buick MK, Bixler EO, et al. Morphology of the uvula in obstructive sleep apnea. Am Rev Respir Dis 1989;140:724–8.

39. Kryger M, Felipe L, Holder D, et al. The sleep deprivation syndrome of the obese patient—a problem of periodic nocturnal upper airway obstruction. Am J Med 1974;56:531–9.

40. Mortimore I, Marshall I, Wraith P, et al. Neck and total body fat deposition in non-obese and obese patients with obstructive sleep apnea compared with that in control subjects. Am J Respir Crit Care Med 1998;157:280–3.

41. Beaumont M, Fodil R, Isabey D, et al. Gravity effects on upper airway area and lung volumes during parabolic flight. J Appl Physiol 1998;84(5):1639–45.

42. Morrison DL, Launois SH, Isono S, et al. Pharyngeal narrowing and closing pressures in patients with obstructive sleep apnea. Am Rev Respir Dis 1993;148:606–11.

43. Isono S, Morrison DL, Launois SH, et al. Static mechanics of the velopharynx of patients with obstructive sleep apnea. J Appl Physiol 1993;75:148–54.

44. Basner RC, Ringler J, Schwartzstein RM, et al. Phasic electromyographic activity of the genioglossus increases in normals during slow-wave sleep. Respir Physiol 1991;83:189–200.

45. Epstein LJ, Kristo D, Strollo PJ Jr, et al, Adult Obstructive Sleep Apnea Task Force of the American Academy of Sleep Medicine. Clinical guideline for the evaluation, management and long-term care of obstructive sleep apnea in adults. J Clin Sleep Med 2009;5(3):263–76.

46. BaHammam A. Excessive daytime sleepiness in patients with sleep disordered breathing. Eur Respir J 2008;31:685–6.

47. Vgontzas AN. Excessive daytime sleepiness in sleep apnea: it is not just apnea hypopnea index. Sleep Med 2008;9:712–4.

48. Oksenberg A, Arons E, Nasser K, et al. Severe obstructive sleep apnea: sleepy versus nonsleepy patients. Laryngoscope 2010;120(3):643–8.

49. Mediano O, Barcelo A, de la Pena M, et al. Daytime sleepiness and polysomnographic variables in sleep apnea patients. Eur Respir J 2007;30:110–3.

50. Roure N, Gomez S, Mediano O, et al. Daytime sleepiness and polysomnography in obstructive sleep apnea patients. Sleep Med 2008;9:727–31.

51. Johns MW. A new method for measuring daytime sleepiness: the Epworth sleepiness scale. Sleep 1991;14:540–5.
52. Samsoon GL, Young JR. Difficult tracheal intubation: a retrospective study. Anaesthesia 1987;42:487–90.
53. Bair AE, Caravelli R, Tyler K, et al. Feasibility of the preoperative Mallampati airway assessment in Emergency Department patients. J Emerg Med 2010;38: 677–80. DOI: 10.1016/j.jemermed.2008.12.019.
54. Kushida CA, Littner MR, Morgenthaler T, et al. Practice parameters for the indications for polysomnography and related procedures: an update for 2005. Sleep 2005;28:499–521.
55. Kushida CA, Morgenthaler TI, Littner MR, et al. Practice parameters for the treatment of snoring and obstructive sleep apnea with oral appliances: an update for 2005. Sleep 2006;29:240–3.
56. Kushida CA, Littner MR, Hirshkowitz M, et al. Practice parameters for the use of continuous and bilevel positive airway pressure devices to treat adult patients with sleep-related breathing disorders. Sleep 2006;29:375–80.
57. Ferguson KA, Cartwright R, Rogers R, et al. Oral appliances for snoring and obstructive sleep apnea: a review. Sleep 2006;29:244–62.
58. SAGES Guidelines Committee. SAGES guideline for clinical application of laparoscopic bariatric surgery. Surg Endosc 2008;22:2281–300.
59. Morgenthaler TI, Kapen S, Lee-Chiong T, et al. Practice parameters for the medical therapy of obstructive sleep apnea. Sleep 2006;29:1031–5.

Index

Note: Page numbers of article titles are in **boldface** type.

A

Abscess
   parapharyngeal, 933–936
   peritonsillar, 932–933
   retropharyngeal, 933–936
Acoustic neuroma, 981, 998
Acoustic reflex, 979
Acrivastine, for allergies, 898
Acute bacterial otitis externa, 962–963
Airway compromise
   for epiglottitis, 937
   sore throat with, 926
Airway management, for pharyngeal abscesses, 934
Alcohol use, cancer related to, 1034–1035
Allergic shiner, 894
Allergies, **891–902**
   classification of, 891
   diagnosis of, 899–900
   epidemiology of, 891
   history in, 892
   hoarseness in, 948–949
   immunotherapy for, 899–900
   symptoms of, 891–896
   treatment of, 896–899
Alveolar nerve, inferior, injury of, in cancer, 1036
Alveolar ridges, cancer of. *See* Cancer, head and neck.
Aminoglycosides, ototoxicity of, 981–982, 998
Amoxicillin, for sinusitis, 887
Antibiotics
   for bacterial pharyngitis, 930
   for epistaxis, 909–910
   for hoarseness, 956
   for mastoiditis, 966
   for otitis externa, 962–963
   for peritonsillar abscess, 932–933
   for pharyngeal abscesses, 935–936
   for sinusitis, 887–888
Antihistamines
   for allergies, 896, 898
   for postnasal drip, 918
Anxiety, dizziness in, 1000

Med Clin N Am 94 (2010) 1057–1074
doi:10.1016/S0025-7125(10)00126-4
0025-7125/10/$ – see front matter © 2010 Elsevier Inc. All rights reserved.

medical.theclinics.com

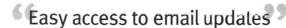

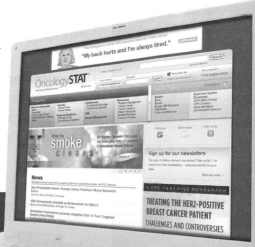